T0407970

CARPAL TUNNEL SYNDROME

RISK FACTORS, SYMPTOMS AND TREATMENT OPTIONS

NEUROANATOMY RESEARCH AT THE LEADING EDGE

Additional books in this series can be found on Nova's website under the Series tab.

Additional e-books in this series can be found on Nova's website under the e-book tab.

NEUROANATOMY RESEARCH AT THE LEADING EDGE

CARPAL TUNNEL SYNDROME

RISK FACTORS, SYMPTOMS AND TREATMENT OPTIONS

MORTON LEDFORD
EDITOR

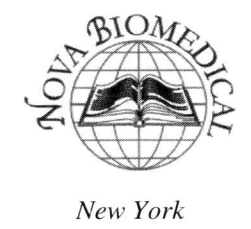

New York

Library of Congress Cataloging-in-Publication Data

ISBN: 978-1-63321-142-1
Library of Congress Control Number: 2014940580

Published by Nova Science Publishers, Inc. † *New York*

Contents

Preface

Carpal tunnel syndrome (CTS) is the most common compressive focal neuropathy of the upper limb. Patients usually have symptoms of numbness, and weakness in the hand, with or without the wrist pain, which may radiate up to the forearm, resulting from compression of the median nerve at the wrist beneath the transverse carpal ligament. The diagnosis is mostly clinical and electrodiagnostic studies are usually performed to confirm the diagnosis and to grade the severity. The most important risk factor for CTS recognized over the years is environmental including repetitive movements of wrist or prolonged positioning of the wrist in extreme flexion or extension position and exposure to vibration. Besides the environmental factors, compression of the nerve can be due to external compression such as a tumor or osteoarthritic changes. Other medical factors that affect the volume of the tunnel also are important risk factors. Treatment of CTS falls under two categories: conservative or surgical. The objective of this book is to provide an overview of carpal tunnel syndrome with emphasis on the risk factors, clinical symptoms and evidence-based overview of treatments options for this common and disabling condition.

Chapter 1 - Carpal Tunnel Syndrome (CTS) is the most common upper extremity neuropathy, accounting for 90% of all entrapment neuropathies. The prevalence of CTS varies from 0.125% to 5.8% of population and the incidence in United States has been estimated to be from 1-3 cases per 1,000. Patients usually present with numbness, and weakness in the hand, with or without the wrist pain, which may radiate up to the forearm, resulting from compression of the median nerve at the wrist beneath the transverse carpal ligament. The diagnosis is mostly clinical and electrodiagnostic studies are usually performed to confirm the diagnosis and to grade the severity. The most important risk factor for CTS recognized over the years is environmental including repetitive movements of wrist or prolonged positioning of the wrist in extreme flexion or extension position and exposure to vibration. Besides the environmental factors, compression of the nerve can be due to external compression such as a tumor or osteoarthritic changes. Other medical factors that affect the volume of the tunnel also are important risk factors. Treatment of CTS falls under two categories: conservative or surgical.

The objective of this review is to provide an overview of carpal tunnel syndrome with emphasis on the risk factors, clinical symptoms and evidence-based overview of treatments options for this common and disabling condition.

Chapter 2 - *Purpose:* To describe the author's experience using the MANOS device for minimally invasive carpal tunnel release.

Methods: The MANOS Carpal Tunnel Release device is a blade that divides the transverse carpal ligament using wrist and palm skin punctures. The awake patient provides feedback as the surgeon navigates a 2.1-mm-diameter blunt probe across the undersurface of the ligament from a wrist incision with ultrasound guidance and/or standard disposable nerve stimulator. The leading tip of the blunt probe is uninsulated and conducts 2 mA. The surgeon converts the blunt insulated probe into an uninsulated blade by advancing a 0.9-mm needle through the palm with a thumb-activated deployment feature. The surgeon saws the ligament from inside out through the 2 skin punctures. Cases were performed with only nerve stimulation in 14 patients, both ultrasound and nerve stimulation method in 12 and only ultrasound guidance in 63 patients. Four had open procedures when ultrasound indicated safe zone for device insertion was too small. Levine Katz validated outcome questionnaires were collected in all patients at three months and 78 patients (84%) at one year.

Results: Symptom severity and functional status scores for patients treated with the MANOS device are comparable to literature controls for endoscopic surgery at 3 months and were improved compared to open surgery controls. Average return to work was 14 days for those working outside the house and 20 days for those with occupational claims. There was one incomplete release. Ninety three percent had good results at one year. Symptom severity and functional status scores at one year were the same as reported by endoscopic and open controls.

Conclusions: Validated outcome scores at three months in patients treated with the MANOS device are comparable to endoscopic results and better than with open surgery. One year results indicate the MANOS Carpal Tunnel

Release device to be safe and effective with regard to definitive healing. Ultrasound was the preferred method for guidance compared to the nerve stimulation method as experience with ultrasound grew.

Chapter 3 - Carpal Tunnel Syndrome (CTS) is known to affect manual dexterity. Electrodiagnostic tests are often used to quantify the extent of damage (mild to severe) of the median nerve. However, these clinical measures of median nerve damage cannot be used to quantify the extent of hand functional deficits. To address this question, several recent studies have been conducted to quantify the behavioral effects of CTS on patients' ability to perform grasping and dexterous manipulation. These studies have used biomechanical analyses to identify functional deficits in hand control due to sub-optimal sensorimotor integration caused by reduced tactile sensitivity at a subset of the digits. The authors review published studies and present novel findings about the effects of CTS on patients' sensorimotor deficits. These deficits are revealed by tasks that require the ability to integrate sensory feedback with motor commands for coordinating digit forces and position. The findings of this research have shown that chronic median nerve compression affects the ability to coordinate preprogrammed and feedback-driven control for effective and efficient force adaptation in multi-digit grasping.

Chapter 4 - Study design. Narrative review of diagnostic studies.

Introduction. Carpal tunnel syndrome (CTS) is one of the most common pathologies of the peripheral nervous system. Several clinical tests have been proposed to diagnose CTS, despite the fact that their psychometric properties continue to be disputed. The aim of this contribution is to collect, through a narrative review of literature, scientific evidence on the accuracy (reliability and validity) of diagnostic tests in CTS, and summarize current knowledge.

Methods. Research was carried out in the main biomedical electronic databases (PubMed, PEDro, EMBASE, CINAHL, Cochrane Library). The following key words were used: "Carpal tunnel syndrome", "Physical examination", "Nerve conduction testing", "Median neuropathy", "Tension test", "Diagnostic testing", with no limits of date and in English, Spanish, Portuguese, French and Italian.

Results. This review concerns the following assessment tools: the Hand Diagram, the Inspection, the Neurological Exam, Tinel's test, Phalen's and Phalen's reverse tests, the Pressure Provocation Tests, the Upper Limb Neurodynamic Tests, and clusters of tests. Other tests such as the Tethered Median Nerve Stress test, the Hand elevation test, the Flick sign, the Closed Fist Sign, and the Tourniquet test are less used in clinical practice. The rates of reliability and diagnostic accuracy of various tests commonly used in CTS appear conflicting.

Conclusion. To make the correct diagnosis, it is advisable to use a cluster of tests rather than a single test. The development of "clinical prediction rules" may be one of the most interesting perspectives for the diagnosis of CTS.

Chapter 5 - Injuries and disease commonly affect the hand and these can significantly affect the ability of an individual to perform activities of daily living. The use of regional outcome measures or scoring systems is important as it allows comparison between these injuries and disease, and allows clinicians to assess progression and the effects of different treatment modalities. A patient-completed questionnaire is efficient in terms of time and resources, and allows the assessment of outcome without the need to attend an outpatient clinic. It is important that the scoring system allows satisfactory regional outcome measurements specific for the hand.

The validity, reliability, responsiveness and bias are used for the assessment of various questionnaires. There are also many practical issues concerning the use of questionnaires including feasibility of use for the patient and the clinician.

The Patient Evaluation Measure (PEM) questionnaire and the Michigan Hand Outcome (MHO) questionnaire are a few of the region-specific outcome measures commonly used for the hand, and are patient-completed questionnaires. They are frequently used to assess self-reported patient outcome in orthopaedics, rheumatology and neurology. In this paper, the validity, reliability, responsiveness and bias of these two questionnaires used for the assessment of the hand will be discussed.

Chapter 6 - Injuries and disease commonly affect the upper limb and these can significantly affect the ability of an individual to perform activities of daily living.

The use of regional outcome measures or scoring systems is important as it allows comparison between these injuries and disease, and allows clinicians to assess progression and the effects of different treatment modalities. A patient-completed questionnaire is efficient in terms of time and resources, and allows the assessment of outcome without the need to attend an outpatient clinic.

It is important that the scoring system allows satisfactory regional outcome measurements specific for the upper limb. This is particularly important in injuries and disease that involve both upper and lower limbs.

The validity, reliability, responsiveness and bias are used for the assessment of various questionnaires. There are also many practical issues concerning the use of questionnaires including feasibility of use for the patient and the clinician.

The Disability of the Arm, Shoulder and Hand (DASH) questionnaire is a region-specific outcome measures commonly used for the upper limb, and is a patient-completed questionnaire. It is frequently used to assess self-reported patient outcome in orthopaedics, rheumatology and neurology. In this paper the DASH questionnaire is discussed along with its disadvantages that lead the authors to create the Manchester-Modified DASH.

With an increasing number of treatment modalities becoming available, and with the emphasis on evidence-based practice, there is an ever-increasing use of regional outcome measures used in the assessment of patients to identify the optimal treatment modality.

These questionnaires are useful as they do not provide limited information about one modality e.g. pain or function, but rather provide a single measure for multiple modalities. It also encompasses a range of symptoms including the physical, social and psychological.

It is important that hand surgeons and other disciplines involved with the care of patients with hand injury and disease have an understanding of the commonly used hand questionnaires.

The Disability of the Arm, Shoulder and Hand (DASH) questionnaire was developed for use in North America (Beaton et al., 2001) but translated versions have been validated in a number of languages including French and Japanese (Imaeda et al., 2005), Spanish (Hervás et al., 2006) and German (Westphal, 2007).

The Disability of the Arm, Shoulder and Hand (DASH) question-naire (Hudak et al., 1996) is probably the most commonly used patient-completed regional outcome measure used for the hand (Khan et al., 2004; Khan and Fahmy, 2006). The main developmental objective was to develop a patient-reported regional outcome measure which considers the upper limb as a single functional unit allowing greater uniformity. The DASH questionnaire measures symptoms and functional status in patients with disorders of the upper limb. It was originally designed and validated as a measure of disability in patients with upper limb disorders.

The DASH questionnaire is used in orthopaedics, rheumatology and neurology to assess self-reported patient outcome (Jupiter and Ring, 2002; McKee et al., 2003).

Chapter 7 - Carpal tunnel syndrome (CTS) is the most frequent mononeuropathy seen in the general population. Defined as median nerve compression at the level of the wrist, CTS causes numbness and tingling in the hand and fingers. The first introduction of the term "carpal tunnel syndrome" is attributed to Brain in 1947 and the popularization of its diagnosis and treatment to Phalen in 1950. Since then, there has been continued debate over the optimal management of this disease. CTS is the most expensive upper-extremity musculoskeletal disorder at an estimated cost of medical care in the US exceeding $2 billion annually, primarily due to surgical releases. The extra-medical costs are substantially greater. In fact, during 2006 in the US, surgeons performed 580,000 outpatient carpal tunnel releases [6] and the median lost work time from work-related CTS is 27 days, which is longer than any other work-related disorder except fractures. Although CTS is a strong driver of workers compensation costs, lost wages, lost productivity, and disability, there is still an in-complete understanding of its frequency and causes in working populations. Prevalent CTS in general populations range from 1–5% and among manufacturing and meat-packing workers has ranged from 5–21%.

Incidence rates from many studies on workers of CTS ranged from 1–15 per 1000 person-years and varied by industrial and occupational. In the general population, the emphasis on possibly risk factors is focused on demographic characteristics (female gender, older age) and on comorbid conditions (higher BMI, rheumatoid arthritis, diabetes mellitus and thyroid disease. Associations between CTS and other risk factors, such as gout, smoking status are uncertain as well as personal and workplace psychosocial possible involvement. However, general population studies do not take workplace exposures into account. The prevalence of CTS in working populations is generally higher than in the general population. Occupation-related CTS represents one of the major health problems among workers in various occupations throughout the world including Sweden, Italy, France, Japan, Taiwan. Recognized occupational risk factors are identify manual loadings with a significantly higher risk or association with CTS, comprise the use of handheld vibrating machinery, forceful gripping of objects with hands, repetitive and frequent manual tasks and forced postures of the wrist (flexion/extension). These loadings are usually combined during occupational work.

Chapter 8 - Injuries and disease commonly affect the ability of an individual to perform activities of daily living. The use of regional outcome measures or scoring systems is important as it allows comparison between these injuries and disease, and allows clinicians to assess progression and the effects of different treatment modalities.

A patient-completed questionnaire is efficient in terms of time and resources, and allows the assessment of outcome without the need to attend an outpatient clinic.

It is important that the scoring system allows satisfactory regional outcome measurements. The validity, reliability, responsiveness and bias are used for the assessment of various questionnaires.

There are also many practical issues concerning the use of questionnaires including feasibility of use for the patient and the clinician. This paper looks at why these measures should be used, their advantages and disadvantages, how they are developed and also how they should be presented. It aims to be useful to those who are developing new questionnaires, as well as those who are using them.

Chapter 9 - Carpal tunnel syndrome (CTS) is a common disorder in hand surgery practice. Both surgical and conservative interventions are utilized for the carpal tunnel syndrome, although certain indications would specifically indicate the need for surgery.

Conservative management is typically preferred for transient cases of CTS such as those associated with pregnancy, short-term overuse or where other exacerbating phenomena are expected to be corrected. In other cases conservative management might be used for partial relief of symptoms while awaiting surgery or for diagnostic purposes in determining patient response [1].

The surgical intervention for CTS is recommended in remaining case, in which is common to find out these characteristics: constant numbness, symptoms > 1 year durations, sensory loss, thenar weakness/atrophy.

The first popularization of diagnosis and treatment of "carpal tunnel syndrome" is attributed to Phalen in 1950. Since then, there has been continued debate over the optimal management of this disease [2]. Currently, surgical options include these techniques: carpal tunnel release with a standard open, carpal tunnel release using various incision techniques (such as mini-open), endoscopic carpal tunnel release, open carpal tunnel release with additional procedures such as internal neurolysis, epineurotomy or tenosynovectomy.

From August 2004 to November 2013, 780 procedures of carpal tunnel release using a mini open incision technique have been performed in our department.

The procedure starts with an accurate skin detersion and disinfection. The intervention have been performed under local anesthesia and exsanguination with pneumatic tourniquet at the limb. The wrist extended approximately 30°.

2 cm long scalpel incision on Taleisnik line. Retraction of skin edges, incision of palmar aponeurosis, exposition and complete opening of flexor retinaculum to perform an external neurolysis of median nerve from fibro/adherential tissue. Before the wound closure a water dissection is performed to complete the procedure and to evaluate the decompression within the carpal tunnel.

Postoperative bulky dressing and skin sutures are kept for 10 days and then removed.

No complications like nerve, vascular or tendon damage, nor infection, relapse or failed treatment occurred. The one exception was a case of postoperative wound infection in a patient who dirtied the dressing during activities in a farm. In all cases patients referred a fast total regression of preoperatively symptoms. No painful and hypertrophic scars were observed.

Chapter 10 - Since Sir James Paget firstly described carpal tunnel syndrome (CTS) in 1854, CTS has been reported the most common compressive neuropathy of the upper extremity. In 1933, Learmonth published firstly surgical release of the transverse carpal ligament by blind surgical treatment and in 1946, Cannon et al. performed the carpal tunnel release for spontaneous CTS firstly. Since then, diagnosis and treatment in CTS has much progressed. Currently, carpal tunnel decompression is the most common operation for peripheral nerves, with more than 586,000 procedures performed in the United States (US), 2006 alone.

The prevalence of clinically and electrophysiologically confirmed CTS is 2.7% (approximately 3% in women and 2% in men) with peak prevalence in women of 55 to 64 years. A few studies have estimated the incidence of CTS, showing large differences between countries. The annual incidence was 324 in women and 125 in men per 100 000 persons in the general population in southern Sweden, and 542 in women and 304 in men per 100,000 persons in the US. In Korea, total clinically and electrophysiologically diagnosed CTS patients were 4.96 and 0.98 per 1,000 person-years, respectively.

The pathophysiology of CTS is associated with compression of the median nerve arising from increased pressure within the carpal tunnel. Incompatibility between decreased space in the carpal tunnel and increased volume of carpal tunnel contents may result in CTS.

CTS can be diagnosed on the basis of patient's history and clinical findings. Some physical examinations are important, but not exclusive for a CTS diagnosis. Advances in scientific tools such as neurophysiological test, MRI and ultrasonography are much helpful in diagnosis, also provided valuable insights into the pathophysiology of CTS.

Treatment of CTS may be selected considering the stage of the disease, the severity of the symptoms, or the preference of the patient. If conservative treatment failed, surgery should be considered, such as conventional open carpal tunnel release (OCTR), mini-OTCR, and endoscopic carpal tunnel release (ETCR).

There has been a variety of surgical techniques for the operative treatment of carpal tunnel syndrome (CTS). Recently, minimally invasive techniques for decompression of the median nerve were developed and introduced such as endoscopic carpal tunnel release (ECTR) and use of a carpal tunnel tome with a small palmar incision. Although many investigators described the advantages of minimally invasive carpal tunnel decompression techniques, numerous cases of iatrogenic injury to the neurovascular structure have been reported. Insufficient anatomical understanding of the carpal tunnel and poor visualization of the surgical field are two major causes of complication during minimally invasive surgery for CTS. In addition, hematoma formation associated with carpal tunnel release may lead to an increased rate of wound infection or delay in wound healing.

To obtain a good surgical outcome for CTS, it is essential to understand the neurovascular anatomy and anatomic variation around the carpal tunnel that these neurovascular structures may take. This chapter will also discuss the anatomical variations and about the changing location of the neurovascular structures during various wrist positions, especially since the wrist position can change unintentionally during surgery using local anesthesia.

In: Carpal Tunnel Syndrome
Editor: Morton Ledford

ISBN: 978-1-63321-142-1
© 2014 Nova Science Publishers, Inc.

Chapter 1

Carpal Tunnel Syndrome: An Overview

Divisha Raheja, M.D. and Aiesha Ahmed[1,], M.D.*

[1]Assistant Professor of Neurology, Penn State Hershey Medical Center,
Department of Neurology, Hershey, PA, US
[2]Assistant Professor of Neurology, Program Director, Clinical
Neurophysiology & Neuromuscular Medicine Fellowships,
Penn State Hershey Medical Center, Department of Neurology,
Hershey, PA, US

Abstract

Carpal Tunnel Syndrome (CTS) is the most common upper extremity neuropathy, accounting for 90% of all entrapment neuropathies. The prevalence of CTS varies from 0.125% to 5.8% of population and the incidence in United States has been estimated to be from 1-3 cases per 1,000. Patients usually present with numbness, and weakness in the hand, with or without the wrist pain, which may radiate up to the forearm, resulting from compression of the median nerve at the wrist beneath the transverse carpal ligament. The diagnosis is mostly clinical and electrodiagnostic studies are usually performed to confirm the diagnosis and to grade the severity. The most important risk factor for CTS recognized over the years is environmental including repetitive

---

[*] Corresponding author. E-mail: aahmed1@Hmc.Psu.Edu.

movements of wrist or prolonged positioning of the wrist in extreme flexion or extension position and exposure to vibration. Besides the environmental factors, compression of the nerve can be due to external compression such as a tumor or osteoarthritic changes. Other medical factors that affect the volume of the tunnel also are important risk factors. Treatment of CTS falls under two categories: conservative or surgical.

The objective of this review is to provide an overview of carpal tunnel syndrome with emphasis on the risk factors, clinical symptoms and evidence-based overview of treatments options for this common and disabling condition.

Introduction

Carpal tunnel syndrome (CTS) is the most common compressive focal neuropathy of the upper limb. The incidence is approximately 7 cases per 10 000 annually. Carpal tunnel release (CTR) usually provides full resolution of symptoms. However, treatment failure and complications are noted in 1% to 25% of all CTR published reports, with a reoperation rate of up to 12%. [1] About 82% of the patients are over 40 years old, and 65%–75% of cases are seen in women. About 50% of the patients may present with bilateral symptoms. It is estimated that up to one-half million surgical releases are performed per year in the United States, with the annual economic cost exceeding $2 billion. [2]

Anatomy of the Carpal Tunnel

The carpal tunnel is a conduit through which nine flexor tendons and the median nerve travels through to enter the hand. The transverse carpal ligament (TCL) is situated volarly, the carpus bone forms the floor and the walls. The width of the tunnel proximally and distally is roughly 25 mm, whereas the narrowest region is at the level of the hamate. The TCL is attached to the scaphoid and trapezium laterally and the hamate and pisiform bones medially. Deep to the TCL, the median nerve is located most superficially, and usually courses just lateral to the midline. The remaining structures within the tunnel include the four tendons of flexor digitorum superficialis and the four tendons of the flexor digitorum profundus muscles, which are encapsulated by the ulnar bursa, and the flexor pollicis longus muscle, which is encapsulated in the radial bursa. [3]

Median nerve

The median nerve comprises of the medial and lateral cords of the brachial plexus, which contain fibers from the sixth, seventh, and eighth cervical and the first thoracic nerve roots. In the upper arm, the median nerve travels with the brachial artery and together they enter the antecubital fossa. Subsequently, the median nerve enters the forearm passing through certain arches. In the forearm, the median nerve gives off anterior interosseus nerve (AIN) branch proximally. At approximately five cm proximal to the wrist crease, the palmar cutaneous branch of the median nerve arises. The median nerve then crosses the wrist, traversing the carpal tunnel to enter the hand. The median nerve goes on to divide into motor and sensory divisions. The motor division supplies the first and second lumbricals, In addition, the recurrent thenar motor branch comes off and supplies the thenar muscles (opponens pollicis, abductor pollicis brevis, and superficial head of flexor pollicis brevis). The sensory division splits to form the common digital nerve to the thumb, common digital nerves of the second and third web spaces and the proper digital nerve to the radial half of the index finger. [4]

Clinical Presentation and Diagnosis

Patients usually complain of numbness and/or paresthesias in the median-nerve distribution, rather than pain. Some patients describe pain as well in the same distribution. These symptoms are typically worse at night and are improved with shaking of the hand, known as the flick sign. Patients may describe discomfort in the thenar eminence. A history of dropping objects correlates with weakness of the opponens pollicis and abductor pollicis brevis muscles. Atrophy of the thenar muscles represents advanced disease. [5] The utility of physical examination has been questioned over time. However, it can still provide some useful information in the diagnosis of CTS. The common provocative tests done during exams are Phalen, Tinel and Durkin carpal compression tests. Phalen is a wrist flexion test. Holding the wrists in maximal flexion for up to 60 seconds reproduces or exacerbates paresthesias or numbness in the median nerve distribution in the hand. Light tapping over the median nerve at the wrist produces similar symptoms in the Tinel test. Similarly, in Durkin test, a direct pressure at or just proximal to the carpal tunnel produces the above mention symptoms. [6]

In all clinically suspected cases, electrodiagnostic studies are recommended. The median sensory nerve distal latencies should be measured on nerve conduction studies (NCS) and compared to either the ulnar or radial sensory latencies in the same hand. Using two comparison techniques that agree (either normal or abnormal) lowers the risk of a false positive or false negative as well as are adequate to confirm the diagnosis. In cases where the testing is borderline, extra testing can help clarify the diagnosis. If the median sensory response is absent, the use of median motor latency in comparison to the ulnar motor latency can help localize the problem. When comparison nerve conduction studies are abnormal for CTS in one limb and that limb is the only symptomatic limb, the American Association of Neuromuscular and Electrodiagnostic Medicine (AANEM) guidelines does not recommend performing NCSs on the opposite hand. If the symptoms are bilateral, or more diffuse, then NCSs on the opposite side are useful. NCSs in the asymptomatic limb are not required to diagnose CTS. These recommendations are part of the practice parameters for electrodiagnostic testing in CTS, and have been published by the AANEM. These also have been incorporated by the American Academy of Orthopedic Surgeons (AAOS) evidence-based guidelines. [7]

Risk Factors

In a recent case–control study by Coggon et al., electrodiagnostically confirmed CTS patients showed association with obesity, work with hand-held vibratory tools, and prolonged repetitive occupational movements of the wrist or fingers, as well as with poor mental health and psychosocial stressors at work. [8] Work related risk factors have been given a great deal of attention. In 2012, an expert committee of the German Ministry for Labor and Social Affairs suggested carpal tunnel syndrome (CTS) as an "occupational disease". Their systematic literature review and meta-analysis was aimed at identifying risk factors for CTS. While trying to address the occupational factors of CTS, manual loading was considered higher risk along with repetition, wrist flexion, powerful grip, and vibration. [9] Interesting, Seror et al., in 2011 had concluded that in patients of working age, the risk of CTS was significantly reduced for white-collar workers using computers. Their results suggested that for workers using computers, computer use could have a direct beneficial effect or a resting effect as it prevents such workers from performing the more strenuous manual tasks performed by blue-collar workers and non-workers. [10]

In a study done by McDairmid et al., it was noted that for the same job task, men and women suffered similar rates of CTS. This study concluded that women are exposed to higher risks for CTS due to their higher concentration in high-risk occupations. For example, in 1990 the study noted that the percentage of women was as follows across different high risk professions: 98.4% of dental hygienists, 94.3% of typists, 93.4% of dressmakers, 90.6% of billing clerks, 89.6% of hairdressers, 89.6% of bookkeepers, and 88.7% of payroll and timekeeping clerks were women. [11]

It is also noted that certain co-morbidities predispose to developing CTS. Examples would be conditions such as metabolic diseases (hyperlipidemia, hyperglycemia and obesity). [12] Similarly, estrogenic status as seen in pregnancy is also considered a risk factor. [13] A multivariate analysis done in UK showed that the risk factors associated with CTS in general community were previous wrist fracture, rheumatoid arthritis, osteoarthritis of the wrist and carpus, obesity, diabetes, and hypothyroidism. Smoking, hormone replacement therapy, the combined oral contraceptive pill and oral corticosteroids were not associated with CTS in this study. [14]

Other rare etiological considerations include masses in or around the median. Both intraneural and extraneural tumors may lead to median nerve compression. Extraneural lesions include lipomas, ganglion cysts, hemangiomas, tenosynovitis, rheumatoid nodules, calcium and uric acid deposits and amyloid infiltration. Tumors involving the peripheral nerves are extremely infrequent as etiology of CTS. The tumors of peripheral nerves are benign in at least 85–90 % of cases and the majority of these tumors are schwannomas. [15]

Differential Diagnosis

This includes cervical radiculopathy, thoracic outlet syndrome, brachial plexopathy, polyneuropathy, strokes, and syringomyelia. In cervical radiculopathy, symptoms can be elicited by passive extension of the neck as well as lateral flexion toward the side of the affected hand. The radial pulse in thoracic outlet syndrome may be extinguished by the Adson maneuver (neck extension and rotation to the ipsilateral side accompanied by deep inspiration). Obtaining a careful history and examination demonstrating neurologic deficits in other nerve distributions can be important in localizing a process to either the central nervous system or brachial plexus. [2]

Management of Carpal Tunnel Syndrome

Treatment of carpal tunnel syndrome has been divided into conservative non surgical options and surgical treatment. Non surgical management is usually reserved for mild to moderate cases and surgical treatment is typically offered to the severe cases or patients with recurrent carpal tunnel syndrome.

Nonsurgical Treatment

Splinting

Splinting involves wearing a splint which immobilizes the wrist in either a neutral position or a slightly extended position. The rationale of benefit from wrist splinting is based on the fact that the symptoms of CTS improve with rest and worsen with activity [16] and compression of the median nerve beneath the transverse ligament, hence immobilizing the wrist in a neutral to 20 degree extension position minimizes the pressure on the carpal tunnel. [17] Patients who use splints at night time have been noted to show improvement in symptoms, hand function and overall improvement in short term. [17] Full time splinting does not offer any additional benefit compared to just night time use. [18] A limited, short term study which looked at the splinting in neutral position when compared to splinting in 20 degree extension has shown neutral position splinting to be slightly superior in improving the overall and nocturnal symptoms relief. [19] Overall, the splinting has been shown to show improvement in short term compared to no treatment, but the latest cochrane review concluded that there is insufficient evidence to suggest long term benefit of splinting and insufficient evidence to suggest any additional benefit compared to other non surgical treatment options. [20] A recent randomized control trial compared the use of night time soft brace with the nighttime splint and showed similar improvement in symptoms in both the groups at three months and did not find any significant difference in favor of either group. [21]

Therapeutic Ultrasound

Ultrasound therapy involves delivery of sound waves to the underlying soft tissues such as ligaments and tendons, producing an anti-inflammatory and tissue stimulating effect by increasing membrane permeability, altering connective tissue excitability and nerve conduction. Ultrasound therapy compared to placebo has been noted to be beneficial for symptom relief in patients with carpal tunnel syndrome after 7 weeks of therapy; no difference in symptoms relief was seen after 2 weeks of therapy. Even after 7 weeks of therapy, no significant difference was noted in the long term nerve conduction studies and grip and pinch strength. [22,23] Different intensities of ultrasound therapy have been compared (1.5W/cm [2] and 0.8 W/cm^2) and no significant difference has been found of one intensity over the other. [23] No significant effect of varying frequency (1 vs. 3 MHz) of ultrasound therapy has been demonstrated on symptom relief or improving function in the short term. [24] There is insufficient evidence to support the therapeutic ultrasound over other non surgical techniques such as splinting, exercises or oral drugs. [25]

Oral Medications

Non steroidal anti-inflammatory drugs (NSAIDs) and diuretics when compared to placebo do not offer any significant relief in short term on the CTS symptoms. [26] Oral steroids have been shown to show overall improvement after short term treatment compared to placebo. There was no difference between the choice of steroids (prednisone or prednisolone). [26–28] The duration of therapy, 2 weeks vs. 4 weeks also did not show any significant difference in the long term benefit. [29,30] Short term steroids when compared to either NSAIDs or the diuretics have shown significant improvement in the CTS symptoms. [31] Lastly, there is no evidence to support the role of vitamin B6 in treatment of CTS in the short term. [32]

Corticosteroid Injections

Local corticosteroid injections have been identified a common and very effective non surgical treatment for patients with CTS. Two high quality, randomized controlled trials reviewed the role of local steroid injections compared to placebo, and showed significant clinical improvement in the short term. [33,34] Compared to systemic corticosteroids, local injections have been noted to be more beneficial, though in short term, no significant difference was noted at 2 weeks and 8 weeks between local steroid injections vs. oral NSAIDs plus wrist splinting. [35] Neither short vs. long acting steroids nor low vs. high dose showed any significant difference in the clinical symptoms. Two local corticosteroid injections do not provide significant added clinical benefit compared to one injection. [35]

Other Non Interventional Therapies

Three randomized control trials have reviewed low level laser therapy compared to placebo and did not find a significant benefit on the outcomes of pain control, hand performance including grip or pinch strength in the short term. [32] Two randomized control trials comparing the ergonomic keyboards vs. standard keyboards have been performed and have failed to reveal any evidence to support the use of ergonomic equipment. [36,37] Magnet therapy has not shown any benefit on pain compared to placebo at 2 weeks; [38] however, moderate evidence has been found in favor of dynamic magnetic field therapy in the short term. [39] There is no clear evidence to support either the chiropractic care or laser acupuncture in treatment of carpal tunnel. [31,32] Yoga has been compared to the wrist splinting and there has been limited evidence that both of these therapies provide similar benefit in nocturnal awakenings, tinel's sign and the grip strength. Short term pain relief was reported better with yoga than the wrist splinting. [40] Lastly, limited evidence has been proven in favor of other exercise and mobilization interventions such as nerve and tendon gliding exercises, carpal bone mobilization and soft tissue mobilization techniques such as massage therapy. [41]

Surgical Treatment

Surgical treatment of CTS is recommended mostly in the severe cases or if the conservative treatment fails. The main goal of the CTS surgery is to minimize the pressure on the median nerve and increase the volume of carpal tunnel by dividing the transverse carpal ligament. CTS surgery can be performed endoscopically or through an open incision.

Endoscopic Carpal Tunnel Release vs. Open Carpal Tunnel Release

Endoscopic carpal tunnel release (ECTR), first described in 1989 is performed with two small incisions proximal or distal to the carpal tunnel. The procedure is performed endoscopically, and the transverse ligament is cut from beneath so as to avoid any damage to the subcutaneous tissue and the skin. Two commonly used techniques are one portal technique described by Agee and the two portal technique described by Chow. [45,46] Most recent cochrane guidelines conclude that ECTR is as effective as open carpal tunnel release in terms of relieving symptoms and improving functional status. No major complications are associated with either procedure, though ECTR is associated with fewer minor complications compared to open surgery and the recovery time is much shorter in patients with ECTR. [47] Rate of recurrence of symptoms and need for repeat surgery are comparable for both procedures.

Open Carpal Tunnel Release (OCTR) vs. Newer Surgical Techniques

Traditionally CTS surgery used to be performed with a long curvilinear palmar incision. [48] In addition to transecting the transverse carpal ligament, epineurotomy and internal neurolysis are performed if there is scar tissue. [49,50] Standard OCTR has been compared with newer, modified shorter incision techniques and minimal differences have been found in regards to relief of symptoms. Significant earlier return to work has been reported in one study, and not in others. OCTR with lengthening of the flexor retinaculum, internal neurolysis and epineurotomy have been compared with the standard OCTR and no significant benefit has been reported with either of these techniques in terms of symptoms severity score and functional status. In conclusion, no clear evidence stands to support these alternative surgical techniques over the standard OCTR and the decision to consider the open vs. endoscopic release is dependent on surgeon's or patient preference. [51]

Surgical Treatment vs. Nonsurgical Treatment

Surgical treatment has been compared to the non-surgical, conservative treatment, and the last cochrane review in 2008 concluded that the surgical treatment relieves CTS symptoms significantly better than splinting, though it still is unclear whether CTS surgery is better than the local corticosteroid injections. [42] A total of 317 patients from 4 randomized controlled trials were included in this review and the pooled estimate favored surgery at 3 and 6 months of follow up. Better clinical improvement was noted with surgery compared to the splinting in 2 of these trials at one year. A recent trial compared surgical treatment with NSAIDs, hand therapy for 6 weeks and if no improvement after therapy, ultrasound therapy for 6 weeks. Significant differences were reported in favor of surgery on the CTS assessment questionnaire on function and symptoms at 6 months and 1 year follow up. [43] Another trial reviewed 3 groups; open surgery, a splint worn 24 hours for 3 months and local steroid plus splint. Significantly better outcomes were noted in the symptom severity score and functional capacity scales in the surgical group. [44]

References

[1] Neuhaus V, Christoforou D, Cheriyan T, Mudgal CS. Evaluation and treatment of failed carpal tunnel release. *Orthop Clin North Am.* 2012;43(4):439–47. doi:10.1016/j.ocl.2012.07.013.

[2] Sternbach G. The carpal tunnel syndrome. *J Emerg Med.* 17(3):519–23. Available at: http://www.ncbi.nlm.nih.gov/pubmed/10338251. Accessed March 3, 2014.

[3] Tosti R, Ilyas AM. Acute carpal tunnel syndrome. *Orthop Clin North Am.* 2012;43(4):459–65. doi:10.1016/j.ocl.2012.07.015.

[4] Demircay E, Civelek E, Cansever T, Kabatas S, Yilmaz C. Anatomic variations of the median nerve in the carpal tunnel: a brief review of the literature. *Turk Neurosurg.* 2011;21(3):388–96. doi:10.5137/1019-5149.JTN.3073-10.1.

[5] Popinchalk SP, Schaffer AA. Physical examination of upper extremity compressive neuropathies. *Orthop Clin North Am.* 2012;43(4):417–30. doi:10.1016/j.ocl.2012.07.011.

[6] Macfarlane DG, Williams TG. Efficacy of provocative tests for diagnosis of carpal tunnel syndrome. *Lancet.* 1990;335(8691):727.

[7] Werner RA, Andary M. Electrodiagnostic evaluation of carpal tunnel syndrome. *Muscle Nerve.* 2011;44(4):597–607. doi:10.1002/mus.22208.

[8] Coggon D, Ntani G, Harris EC, et al. Differences in risk factors for neurophysiologically confirmed carpal tunnel syndrome and illness with similar symptoms but normal median nerve function: a case-control study. *BMC Musculoskelet Disord.* 2013;14:240. doi:10.1186/1471-2474-14-240.

[9] Spahn G, Wollny J, Hartmann B, Schiele R, Hofmann GO. [Metaanalysis for the evaluation of risk factors for carpal tunnel syndrome (CTS) Part II. Occupational risk factors]. *Z Orthop Unfall.* 2012;150(5):516–24. doi:10.1055/s-0032-1315346.

[10] Seror P, Seror R. Hand workload, computer use and risk of severe median nerve lesions at the wrist. *Rheumatology (Oxford).* 2012;51(2):362–7. doi:10.1093/rheumatology/ker372.

[11] McDiarmid M, Oliver M, Ruser J, Gucer P. Male and female rate differences in carpal tunnel syndrome injuries: personal attributes or job tasks? *Environ Res.* 2000;83(1):23–32. doi:10.1006/enrs.2000.4042.

[12] Onder B, Yalçın E, Selçuk B, Kurtaran A, Akyüz M. Carpal tunnel syndrome and metabolic syndrome co-occurrence. *Rheumatol Int.* 2013;33(3):583–6. doi:10.1007/s00296-012-2417-1.

[13] Khosrawi S, Maghrouri R. The prevalence and severity of carpal tunnel syndrome during pregnancy. *Adv Biomed Res*. 2012;1:43. doi:10.4103/2277-9175.100143.

[14] Geoghegan JM, Clark DI, Bainbridge LC, Smith C, Hubbard R. Risk factors in carpal tunnel syndrome. *J Hand Surg Br*. 2004;29(4):315–20. doi:10.1016/j.jhsb.2004.02.009.

[15] Dailiana ZH, Bougioukli S, Varitimidis S, et al. Tumors and tumor-like lesions mimicking carpal tunnel syndrome. *Arch Orthop Trauma Surg*. 2014;134(1):139–44. doi:10.1007/s00402-013-1901-8.

[16] Roaf R, Adderley D, Harris HA. Compression of median nerve in carpal tunnel. *Lancet*. 1947;1(6447):387. Available at: http://www.ncbi.nlm.nih.gov/pubmed/20289882. Accessed March 3, 2014.

[17] Manente G, Torrieri F, Di Blasio F, Staniscia T, Romano F, Uncini A. An innovative hand brace for carpal tunnel syndrome: a randomized controlled trial. *Muscle Nerve*. 2001;24(8):1020–5. Available at: http://www.ncbi.nlm.nih.gov/pubmed/11439376. Accessed February 7, 2014.

[18] Walker WC, Metzler M, Cifu DX, Swartz Z. Neutral wrist splinting in carpal tunnel syndrome: a comparison of night-only versus full-time wear instructions. *Arch Phys Med Rehabil*. 2000;81(4):424–9. doi:10.1053/mr.2000.3856.

[19] Burke DT, Burke MM, Stewart GW, Cambré A. Splinting for carpal tunnel syndrome: in search of the optimal angle. *Arch Phys Med Rehabil*. 1994;75(11):1241–4. Available at: http://www.ncbi.nlm.nih.gov/pubmed/7979936. Accessed March 4, 2014.

[20] Page M, Massy-Westropp N, O'Connor D, Pitt V. Splinting for carpal tunnel syndrome (Review). *Cochrane Database Syst Rev*. 2012;(7). Available at: http://onlinelibrary.wiley.com/doi/10.1002/14651858.CD010003/pdf/standard. Accessed March 2, 2014.

[21] De Angelis M V, Pierfelice F, Di Giovanni P, Staniscia T, Uncini A. Efficacy of a soft hand brace and a wrist splint for carpal tunnel syndrome: a randomized controlled study. *Acta Neurol Scand*. 2009;119(1):68–74. doi:10.1111/j.1600-0404.2008.01072.x.

[22] Ebenbichler GR, Resch KL, Nicolakis P, et al. Ultrasound treatment for treating the carpal tunnel syndrome: randomised "sham" controlled trial. *BMJ*. 1998;316(7133):731–5. Available at: http://www.pubmedcentral.nih.gov/articlerender.fcgi?artid=28476&tool=pmcentrez&rendertype=abstract. Accessed March 5, 2014.

[23] Oztas O, Turan B, Bora I, Karakaya MK. Ultrasound therapy effect in carpal tunnel syndrome. *Arch Phys Med Rehabil*. 1998;79(12):1540–4. Available at: http://www.ncbi.nlm.nih.gov/pubmed/9862296. Accessed March 5, 2014.

[24] Koyuncu H, Unver FN, Sahin U TP. 1Mhz - 3MHz ultrasound applications in carpal tunnel syndrome. *Fiz Tedavi ve Rehabil Derg*. 1995;19:141–5.

[25] Mj P, Connor OD, Pitt V. Therapeutic ultrasound for carpal tunnel syndrome (Review). *Cochrane Database Syst Rev*. 2013;(3).

[26] Chang MH, Chiang HT, Lee SS, Ger LP, Lo YK. Oral drug of choice in carpal tunnel syndrome. *Neurology*. 1998;51(2):390–3. Available at: http://www.ncbi.nlm.nih.gov/pubmed/9710008. Accessed March 5, 2014.

[27] Herskovitz S, Berger AR, Lipton RB. Low-dose, short-term oral prednisone in the treatment of carpal tunnel syndrome. *Neurology*. 1995;45(10):1923–5. Available at: http://www.ncbi.nlm.nih.gov /pubmed/7477994. Accessed March 5, 2014.

[28] Hui AC, Wong SM, Wong KS, et al. Oral steroid in the treatment of carpal tunnel syndrome. *Ann Rheum Dis*. 2001;60(8):813–4. Available at: http://www.pubmedcentral.nih.gov/articlerender.fcgi?artid= 1753810&tool=pmcentrez&rendertype=abstract. Accessed March 5, 2014.

[29] Chang M-H, Ger L-P, Hsieh PF, Huang S-Y. A randomised clinical trial of oral steroids in the treatment of carpal tunnel syndrome: a long term follow up. *J Neurol Neurosurg Psychiatry*. 2002;73(6):710–4. Available at: http://www.pubmedcentral.nih.gov/articlerender.fcgi?artid=1757344 &tool=pmcentrez&rendertype=abstract. Accessed March 5, 2014.

[30] Graham BA. Two weeks of prednisolone was as effective as four weeks in improving carpal tunnel syndrome symptoms. *J Bone Joint Surg Am*. 2003;85-A(8):1624. Available at: http://www.ncbi.nlm.nih.gov/pubmed/ 12925658. Accessed March 5, 2014.

[31] O'Connor D. Non-surgical treatment (other than steroid injection) for carpal tunnel syndrome. *Cochrane Database Syst Rev*. 2003;(1). Available at: http://onlinelibrary.wiley.com/doi/10.1002/ 14651858. CD003219/pdf/standard. Accessed March 2, 2014.

[32] Huisstede BM, Hoogvliet P, Randsdorp MS, Glerum S, van Middelkoop M, Koes BW. Carpal tunnel syndrome. Part I: effectiveness of nonsurgical treatments--a systematic review. *Arch Phys Med Rehabil*. 2010;91(7):981–1004. doi:10.1016/j.apmr.2010.03.022.

[33] Dammers JW, Veering MM, Vermeulen M. Injection with methylprednisolone proximal to the carpal tunnel: randomised double blind trial. *BMJ*. 1999;319(7214):884–6. Available at: http://www.pubmedcentral.nih.gov/articlerender.fcgi?artid=28242&tool=pmcentrez&rendertype=abstract. Accessed March 6, 2014.

[34] Armstrong T, Devor W, Borschel L, Contreras R. Intracarpal steroid injection is safe and effective for short-term management of carpal tunnel syndrome. *Muscle Nerve*. 2004;29(1):82–8. doi:10.1002/mus.10512.

[35] Marshall S, Tardif G, Ashworth N. Local corticosteroid injection for carpal tunnel syndrome (Review). *Cochrane Database Syst ...*. 2007;(2). Available at: http://onlinelibrary.wiley.com/doi/10.1002/14651858.CD001554. pub2/pdf/standard. Accessed March 2, 2014.

[36] Connor OD, Mj P, Sc M. Ergonomic positioning or equipment for treating carpal tunnel syndrome (Review). *Cochrane Database Syst Rev*. 2012;(1).

[37] Buchan S, Amirfeyz R. Cochrane corner: ergonomic positioning or equipment for treating carpal tunnel syndrome. *J Hand Surg Eur Vol*. 2013;38(5):580–1. doi:10.1177/1753193413478507.

[38] Carter R, Aspy CB, Mold J. The effectiveness of magnet therapy for treatment of wrist pain attributed to carpal tunnel syndrome. *J Fam Pract*. 2002;51(1):38–40. Available at: http://www.ncbi.nlm.nih.gov/pubmed/11927062. Accessed March 6, 2014.

[39] Weintraub MI, Cole SP. A randomized controlled trial of the effects of a combination of static and dynamic magnetic fields on carpal tunnel syndrome. *Pain Med*. 2008;9(5):493–504. Available at: http://www.ncbi.nlm.nih.gov/pubmed/18777606. Accessed March 6, 2014.

[40] Garfinkel MS, Singhal A, Katz WA, Allan DA, Reshetar R, Schumacher HR. Yoga-based intervention for carpal tunnel syndrome: a randomized trial. *JAMA*. 1998;280(18):1601–3. Available at: http://www.ncbi.nlm.nih.gov/pubmed/9820263. Accessed March 6, 2014.

[41] Page M, O'connor D, Pitt V, Massy-Westropp N. Exercise and mobilisation interventions for carpal tunnel syndrome (Review). *Cochrane Database Syst Rev*. 2012;(6). Available at: http://onlinelibrary.wiley.com/doi/10.1002/14651858.CD009899/pdf/standard. Accessed March 2, 2014.

[42] Rj V, Ra S, Jl C, Jg C. Surgical versus non-surgical treatment for carpal tunnel syndrome (Review). *Cochrane Database Syst Rev*. 2008;(4).

[43] Jarvik JG, Comstock BA, Kliot M, et al. Surgery versus non-surgical therapy for carpal tunnel syndrome: a randomised parallel-group trial. *Lancet.* 2009;374(9695):1074–81. doi:10.1016/S0140-6736(09)61517-8.

[44] Ucan H, Yagci I, Yilmaz L, Yagmurlu F, Keskin D, Bodur H. Comparison of splinting, splinting plus local steroid injection and open carpal tunnel release outcomes in idiopathic carpal tunnel syndrome. *Rheumatol Int.* 2006;27(1):45–51. doi:10.1007/s00296-006-0163-y.

[45] Agee JM, McCarroll HR, North ER. Endoscopic carpal tunnel release using the single proximal incision technique. *Hand Clin.* 1994;10(4):647–59. Available at: http://www.ncbi.nlm.nih.gov/ pubmed/7868632. Accessed March 8, 2014.

[46] Chow JC. The Chow technique of endoscopic release of the carpal ligament for carpal tunnel syndrome: four years of clinical results. *Arthroscopy.* 1993;9(3):301–14. Available at: http://www. ncbi.nlm.nih.gov/pubmed/8323616. Accessed March 8, 2014.

[47] Hs V, Georgoulas P, Shrier I, Salanti G, Rjpm S. Endoscopic release for carpal tunnel syndrome (Review). *Cochrane Database Syst Rev.* 2014;(1).

[48] Taleisnik J. The palmar cutaneous branch of the median nerve and the approach to the carpal tunnel. An anatomical study. *J Bone Joint Surg Am.* 1973;55(6):1212–7. Available at: http://www.ncbi.nlm.nih.gov/ pubmed/4758035. Accessed March 8, 2014.

[49] Fissette J, Onkelinx A. Treatment of carpal tunnel syndrome. Comparative study with and without epineurolysis. *Hand.* 1979;11(2):206–10. Available at: http://www.ncbi.nlm.nih.gov/ pubmed/488797. Accessed March 8, 2014.

[50] Curtis RM, Eversmann WW. Internal neurolysis as an adjunct to the treatment of the carpal-tunnel syndrome. *J Bone Joint Surg Am.* 1973;55(4):733–40. Available at: http://www.ncbi.nlm.nih.gov/ pubmed/4283745. Accessed March 8, 2014.

Rjpm S, A MVDM, Bmj U, Lm B, Hcw DV. Surgical treatment options for carpal tunnel syndrome (Review). *Cochrane Database Syst Rev.* 2007;(4).

In: Carpal Tunnel Syndrome
Editor: Morton Ledford

ISBN: 978-1-63321-142-1
© 2014 Nova Science Publishers, Inc.

Chapter 2

Carpal Tunnel Release Using the MANOS CTR System

Bruce McCormack, M.D.
Clinical Faculty, University of California, San Francisco, CA, US

Abstract

Purpose: To describe the author's experience using the MANOS device for minimally invasive carpal tunnel release.

Methods: The MANOS Carpal Tunnel Release device is a blade that divides the transverse carpal ligament using wrist and palm skin punctures. The awake patient provides feedback as the surgeon navigates a 2.1-mm-diameter blunt probe across the undersurface of the ligament from a wrist incision with ultrasound guidance and/or standard disposable nerve stimulator. The leading tip of the blunt probe is uninsulated and conducts 2 mA. The surgeon converts the blunt insulated probe into an uninsulated blade by advancing a 0.9-mm needle through the palm with a thumb-activated deployment feature. The surgeon saws the ligament from inside out through the 2 skin punctures. Cases were performed with only nerve stimulation in 14 patients, both ultrasound and nerve stimulation method in 12 and only ultrasound guidance in 63 patients. Four had open procedures when ultrasound indicated safe zone for device insertion was too small. Levine Katz validated outcome questionnaires were collected in all patients at three months and 78 patients (84%) at one year.

Results: Symptom severity and functional status scores for patients treated with the MANOS device are comparable to literature controls for endoscopic surgery at 3 months and were improved compared to open surgery controls. Average return to work was 14 days for those working outside the house and 20 days for those with occupational claims. There was one incomplete release. Ninety three percent had good results at one year. Symptom severity and functional status scores at one year were the same as reported by endoscopic and open controls.

Conclusions: Validated outcome scores at three months in patients treated with the MANOS device are comparable to endoscopic results and better than with open surgery. One year results indicate the MANOS Carpal Tunnel Release device to be safe and effective with regard to definitive healing. Ultrasound was the preferred method for guidance compared to the nerve stimulation method as experience with ultrasound grew.

Introduction

Carpal tunnel syndrome (CTS) is the most common entrapment neuropathy [1-6]. It presents with hand pain, numbness and tingling [7-8]. When conservative measures fail, surgery provides predictable relief if the diagnosis is correct and the ligament is completely transected.

The vast majority of carpal tunnel release (CTR) surgeries are performed using an open surgical technique with a palm incision [9-11]. It is a successful procedure, but palm incisions have short term and long term morbidity. This includes delay in returning to activities of daily living and work and persistent pain and tenderness of the cicatrix [12-14].

In an effort to reduce a surgical trauma, endoscopic techniques have been used with success [15]. Adoption is repressed by a steep alerting curve and the fact that endoscopic procedures usually entail higher capital costs, longer operative room setup, and higher complications compared with open surgery [4, 15-16]. Other surgeons advocate mini open incisions [17-18].

Ultrasound (US) has been used as an adjunctive tool for diagnosis of CTS, particularly for patients being evaluated for incomplete release after carpal tunnel surgery and for identifying space occupying lesions [19]. US is commonly used to guide carpal tunnel steroid injections [19-21]. There has also been interest in the use of US to navigate surgical instruments in carpal tunnel surgery. In 1997, Nakamichi reported the first clinical experience with US-guided CTR. His series showed good results in 50 patients and 50 hands using a hybrid technique, opening the distal ligament with open surgery and the proximal ligament with US guidance [22]. Nakamichi reported the second series using a purely percutaneous approach [23].

The MANOS CTR device allows for a minimally invasive technique to be performed in an awake patient using ultrasound to navigate the carpal tunnel from wrist to palm. The cutting device is deployed when the device is positioned satisfactorily. US was used to identify the safe zone for device insertion, for navigation around the tendons, superficial palmar arch, median nerve, ulnar artery and for confirmation of ligament release. The MANOS CTR device is also compatible for use with commercially available nerve stimulators.

This chapter reviews the author's experience using MANOS carpal tunnel blade, with emphasis on surgical technical and outcome analysis with the symptom, severity and functional status validated questionnaire formulated by Levine et al. [24].

Materials and Methods

Between June 2011 and December 2013, the author offered 93 patients a minimally invasive CTR procedure using the MANOS device. The author had acquired approval from the hospital's institutional review board and informed patients of the intent to obtain clinical data for informed consent. These patients were prospectively followed for one year.

All patients had carpal tunnel syndrome by history, examination, and the presence of positive nerve conduction studies. The only exclusion criterion was prior carpal tunnel surgery on the affected hand. We noted associated medical conditions and documented preoperative and postoperative work status. Collected data included the operative report and follow up office notes, looking for residual signs, symptoms and complications. Patients were re-evaluated at two days, two weeks, three months and one year after surgery.

The patients filled out a self-administered, symptom severity and functional status questionnaire by Levine three months and one year after surgery [24]. We calculated the median's course for symptom severity and functional status and compared them with literature controls.

Device

The MANOS device is a CTR blade 2.1 mm in diameter, enclosed in a blunt protective tube. The blade and outer tube are attached to a plastic handle. MANOS device is inserted in the body in a blunt configuration. The saw blade has a unidirectional cutting surface and remains protected by the outer blunt tube until proper positioning is achieved. The blade is then deployed using a thumb slide on the handle which simultaneously ejects a 19 gauge needle through the tip of the outer tube (Figures 1 – 2).

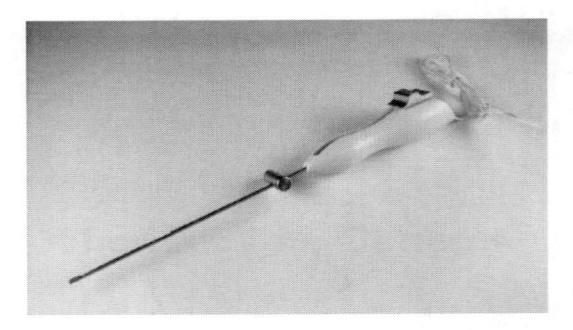

Figure 1. The MANOS CTR device is blunt when inserted into the carpal tunnel. Two milliamps is conducted through the leading tip using a commercially available nerve stimulator.

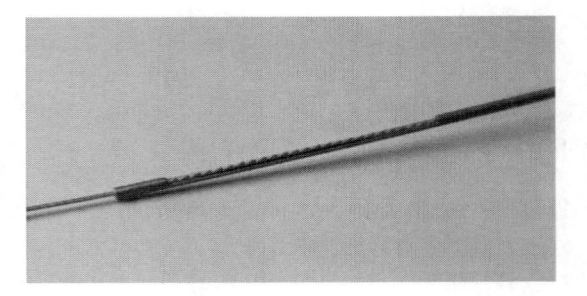

Figure 2. View of the blade exposed on a palmar-directed window on the MANOS device. The unidirectional blade cuts when pulled proximally. The surgeon engages the transverse carpal ligament with the blade by applying pressure on the device against the undersurface of the ligament while simultaneously applying counter pressure on the overlying palm with the other hand.

Operative Procedure

All procedures took place in a standard operating room. The symptomatic hand was positioned on an adjustable sterile board that extended the wrist and abducted the thumb. The proximal arm, fingers and thumb were secured with Velcro straps to free up the surgeon's non-operative hand. We did not use a tourniquet or general anesthesia because patient feedback was necessary for intraoperative assessment of median nerve function.

In the initial 50 patients using the MANOS device, nerve stimulation technique was the primary tool to navigate the wrist. Ultrasound was adjunctive to nerve stimulation technique. With experience, surgeons became more comfortable visualizing anatomy with the ultrasound and the majority stopped using nerve stimulation altogether.

Prior to skin incision, ultrasonography was performed using a high frequency 10 MHz transducer (Sonosite, Bothell, Washington, D.C.) positioned transversely at the level of the hook of the hamate and the tubercle of the trapezius to identify the tunnel. The US transducer was translated distally and proximally to scan the carpal tunnel and its contents, including the median nerve and flexor tendons and proper left-to-right orientation was confirmed. The ulnar artery and nerve and Guyon's canal were identified. Next, the transverse carpal ligament was visualized and followed from proximally to distally to identify the extent of the carpal tunnel and the superficial palmar arterial arch. The median nerve was identified on the basis of the several features. The median nerve, as all nerves, had a distinctive speckled hypoechoic fascicular pattern when visualized along its short axis. In contrast to tendons that exhibit significant anisotropy (appear alternately dark and light) as the transducer was skipped proximally and distally, the median nerve changed little in appearance. The nerve was seen superficially to the flexor tendons and just under the transverse carpal ligament, typically just above the ulnar to the flexor pollicis longus tendon, which could be identified by actively and passively flexing the patient's thumb.

Asking the patient to flex and extend the fingers and thumb while extending the distal wrist at the level of the proximal opening of the carpal tunnel revealed tendon movements perpendicular to the axis of the transducer and along the long axis of the wrist, while the median nerve moved slightly side to side or appeared relatively stationary. Within the carpal tunnel, flattening and reduced motion of the median nerve were often visualized and were consistent with nerve compression.

We infiltrated 2% Lidocaine with 4-8 mL Epinephrine over the transverse carpal ligament. We took care not to anesthetize the median nerve and check its normal function before proceeding.

The entering position point of the MANOS CTR device was 2 cm proximal to the distal wrist crease, just ulnar to the palmaris longus. Figure 3 shows the standard anatomic landmarks that we identified.

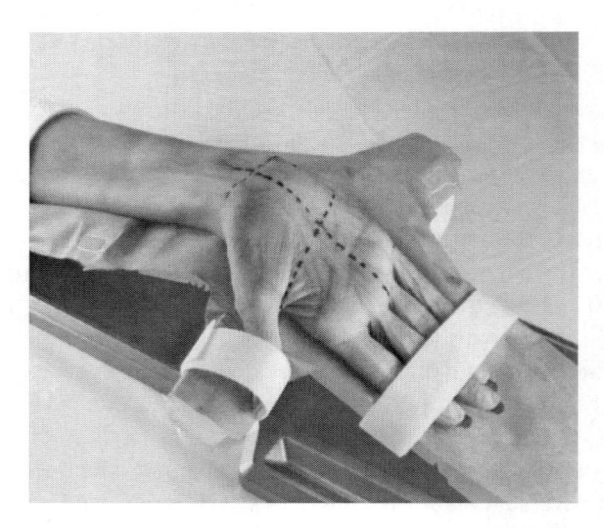

Figure 3. The hand is marked for surgery using well-known surface anatomical landmarks. Entry and exit points are defined, in line with the web of the long and ring fingers. The cardinal line of Kaplan is marked to identify the distal aspect of the transverse carpal ligament.

The safe zone from the median nerve to the hook of hamate typically measured 5-10 mm on US. We made a small skin and fascia incision at the wrist and passed a 3 mm blunt metal probe dilator under the transverse carpal ligament in line with the web of the long and ring fingers. We palpated the undersurface of the transverse carpal ligament with the metal probe for characteristic washboard ridging. The desired trajectory was to skim the undersurface of the ligament and not plunge between tendons. The probe was palpated in the palm in the subcutaneous tissue just distal to the ligament in line with the web of the third and fourth fingers. As experience with US guidance grew, the exact location of the device entry and exit points were slightly modified using patient specific landmarks. We marked entry and exit points before surgery. The finger should move freely, and thumb, finger sensation and strength testing were performed to ensure tendons and median nerve was not snagged by the probe. The probe dissected the synovium and created a track for the MANOS device.

We removed the metal probe and inserted the MANOS device through the track. The device went under the transverse carpal ligament and was advanced in a straight pathway abutting the transverse carpal tunnel ligament, ending up in the subcutaneous tissue at the pre-determined exit point.

Any resistance while advancing the device alerted the surgeon that the device was in subcutaneous tissues and not in the tunnel.

Once the device was satisfactorily positioned, upward pressure from the MANOS device was placed on the deep surface of the transverse carpal ligament. Downward pressure using the free hand was placed on the ligament from the palm to engage the MANOS device. Tendon and nerve checks were repeated. Nerve impingement would result in numbness, tingling or pain in the median nerve distribution. Entrapment of a flexor tendon would limit finger excursion.

We then activated the device by advancing a 0.9 mm needle through the palm just distal to the transverse carpal ligament at the cardinal line of Kaplan. Activation of the device exposed a unidirectional blade through a palmar directed window. A needle exit more distal to the Kaplan line was redirected to the line to prevent injury to the superficial palmar arch, and median and ulnar nerve communicating branches. US was used again to confirm proper placement of the MANOS CTR device. We capped the needle exiting the palm for safety. The adjustable blade lock was secured to prevent the blunt tip of the device from exiting the palmar skin.

The physician then transected the ligament by applying downward pressure on the ligament with one hand and moving the MANOS CTR device in the back and forth motion with the other. The blade cuts when pulled proximally. It operates like a small saw blade—small back and forth excursions of a few centimeters transected the ligament in five to 15 passes depending on ligament thickness. The 0.9 mm needle that exited the palm tracks the cutting tool.

The surgeon's other hand was placed on the skin overlying the ligament, and fingertip pressure was placed for tactile feedback and optimal blade engagement with the transverse carpal ligament. As the device released the ligament, it pulled up into subcutaneous tissues and was palpated with the surgeon's other hand.

The device was visualized in subcutaneous tissues above the transverse carpal ligament via US, confirming complete ligament release (Figure 4).

The safety cap that was placed on the needle exiting the palm was removed, and the blade was retracted into the device assembly. The device was removed through the wrist puncture site.

The blunt metal probe was inserted to palpate the TC ligament and ensure complete release. This final step was added after a case of incomplete release.

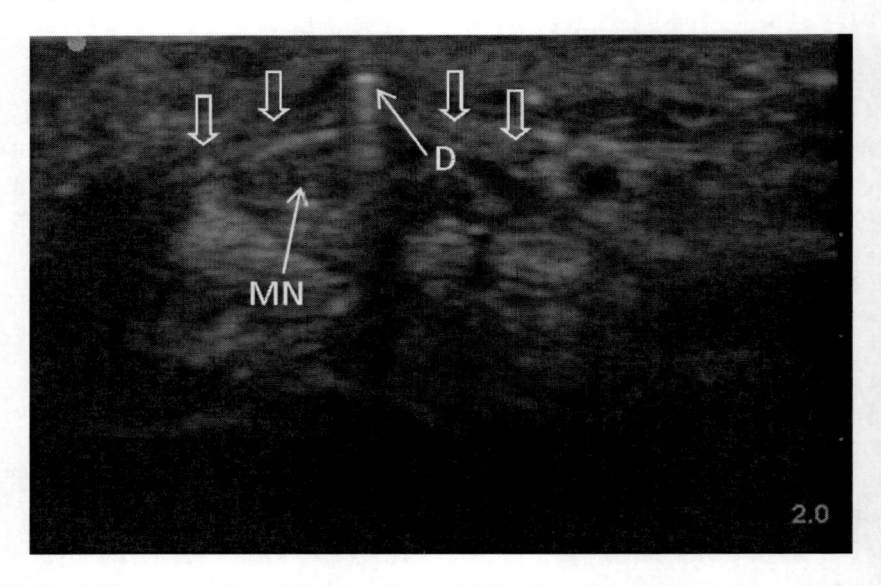

Figure 4. Transverse view of the carpal tunnel following release of transverse carpal ligament, intraoperative image. Transverse carpal ligament, open arrows; median nerve, MN; MANOS CTR device, D.

A tissue adhesive was placed over the palm and wrist puncture sites. A wound dressing was applied. The technique took, on average, ten minutes to complete.

Results

A total of 89 patients who had the MANOS carpal tunnel release and four patients with open release completed a validated symptom severity and functional status questionnaire at three months. One year follow-up was on 78 patients (87%).

Patient age average was 73 (range 39-93 years); 72 patients were women and 21 were men. Preoperative symptoms were present for two to 300 months.

Twenty five patients had diabetes, 29 osteoarthritis, twenty had cervical stenosis with myelopathy (6) and radiculopathy (14), seventeen were obese, fifteen had hypothyroidism, seven had autoimmune disorders and four each had neuropathy, three prior fracture, one renal disease one a prior CRPS.

A total of 33 patients (35%) were employed outside the home before surgery. Of which, sixteen had occupational claims.

Twenty-one had prior carpal tunnel surgery on the other hand using the open approach.

We performed 104 procedures on 93 patients. Four had simultaneous bilateral procedures and another seven had a second procedure for the other hand.

Four patients were converted to open surgery after intraoperative ultrasound prior to incision indicated a high proximal bifurcation of the median nerve (1) and three with inadequate safe zone to insert the device.

There were no vessel or tendon injuries.

Table 1 shows the symptom severity and functional status sores at three months and one year. Literature controls are also presented for comparison.

Table 1. The symptom severity and functional status sores at three months and one year

Study Author	Study Type	Technique	Patients (n)	3 Months Postoperative		12 Months Postoperative	
				Symptom Severity	Functional Status	Symptom Severity	Functional Status
McCormack	Prospective	MANOS CTR®	89	1.7 ± 0.1	6.7 ± 0.3	1.5 ± 0.2	1.5 ± 0.1
Trumble	Prospective	Open	72	2.5 ± 0.1	2.8 ± 0.1	1.8 ± 0.1	1.7 ± 0.1
		Endoscopic	75	1.8 ± 0.1	1.7 ± 0.1	1.8 ± 0.2	1.7 ± 0.1
Atrochi	Prospective	Endoscopic	63	1.5	1.3	1.4	1.3

Average return to work was 14 days and in 18 days in the patients with occupational claims.

Nine patients had minor wound issues. Six had inadvertent skin lacerations at the entry and exit point. Skin lacerations occurred in elderly patients with atrophic skin. All were less than a centimeter and healed uneventfully.

Seven patients had poor outcomes. Four had concurrent cervical spinal stenosis treated with neck surgery and poor outcome was attributed to "double crush". Two patients reported more pain but declined further evaluation and treatment. One of these patients had complex regional pain syndrome after an industrial low back injury and developed RSD like symptoms after open carpal tunnel release. Repeat electrical studies were improved and ultrasound showed complete release. No additional surgery was offered.

There was one case of increased index finger numbness and chronic pain. A 45 year old fireman had simultaneous bilateral procedures using nerve stimulation technique for navigation. Ultrasound was used but it was early in the author's experience. Results of right hand were excellent; left hand results were poor with new index finger numbness and persistent incisional pain with positive Tinel sign. Nerve conduction studies were slightly improved. Ultrasound and MRI were indeterminate. One year after first surgery, wound exploration was performed with scar tissue identified around the median nerve. Results of neurolysis were poor.

One patient had persistent hand numbness and tingling after surgery and had open exploration within a month. Findings were incomplete release of the transverse carpal tunnel ligament. They improved with second surgery. After this case, technique was changed. A probe was passed through the decompression at conclusion of the decompression to confirm release with manual palpation and with an ultrasound image.

Conclusion

Carpal tunnel surgery is safe and effective when the diagnosis is correct and the surgeon accomplishes complete release of the transverse carpal tunnel ligament. Long term overall satisfaction rates are reported at 87% [25]. The vast majority of patients in the United States are treated with open palm incision using a scalpel.

Palm incisions have been associated with persistent pain, tenderness and delay in return to work and activities of daily living [12-14]. Most surgeons agree that minimizing surgical wounds benefits patients as long the intended goal of surgery i.e. sectioning the TCL is not compromised.

There have also been multiple efforts to improve upon results of standard open carpal tunnel surgery using smaller incisions. To date, most advances in minimally invasive carpal tunnel surgery have been endoscopes developed in the 1990's [26] followed by minimal incremental innovation over the past 20 years. Endoscopic techniques have been used with some success but adoption has been hampered because the learning curve remains high, and additional complications have been reported such as neuropraxia and incomplete ligament release [12-18, 24-26].

The MANOS device consisting of a 2.1 mm blunt probe that converts to a cutting device when properly positioned in an awake patient under the transverse carpal ligament. Careful attention to surface landmarks for device entrance and exit make the procedure safe. Entrance point is at the safe zone between the median nerve and ulnar artery. Exit point in the palm just distal to the TCL. Nerve injury is a potential complication if the exit puncture is too distal in the palm. Superficial palmar vascular arch and, more important, ulnar and medial nerve palmar communicating branches [27-28] are at risk for injury with distal palm incisions using both open [29] and endoscopic techniques [30].

Our first publication and experience with the MANOS device was using intraoperative nerve stimulation technique. [31]. Nerve locators have been extensively used to improve safety and minimize surgical morbidity [32-34]. Anesthesiologists use electrical stimulation to advance needles close to, but not contacting, nerve for safe regional blocks [35]. The premise behind the nerve stimulation method is that a motor response occurs before needle to nerve physical contact occurs owing to a zone of depolarization surrounding the needle. The intensity of current needed to produce a motor twitch is inversely proportional to the square of the needle tip nerve distance. Insulated needles that minimize current dispersion provide better accuracy [36]. The initial MANOS device was insulated with a Polymer, except for the leading top edge and saw blade, which were uninsulated and electrically stimulated by attaching the device to a Vari-Stim III nerve locator (Vari-Stim III hand held nerve locator/stimulator; Medtronic Xomed, Jacksonville, Florida) set at 2 mA. We used the highest setting to maximize the opportunity to identify adjacent nerve tissue. The saw blade cuts the transverse carpal ligament incrementally and is not all or none, as with the past with an endoscopic scalpel blade. Incremental saw cuts and the zone of depolarization surrounding the uninsulated saw gives the surgeon opportunity to stop if a nerve response is elicited. While we had good results in our first 50 patients, adoption was suppressed because surgeons considered it a blind procedure and were unfamiliar with nerve stimulation technique. There was concern that a compromised median nerve may not reliably respond to nerve stimulation.

Ultrasound is another available option to provide real time visualization. Initial reports of minimally invasive US-guided CTR suggest advantages over current "mini open" techniques at six and 13 weeks. Nakamichi et al. reported the US guided percutaneous CTR results in superior pain, function, and patient satisfaction scores [23]. In our first series of 50 patients ultrasound was used as an adjunctive technique. But as experience grew, surgeons began to use it as the primary navigation tool.

US is an excellent imaging modality for soft tissue musculoskeletal structures and nerves in particular. Kamolz et al. reported a high correlation of US images with anatomic dissection findings [37]. US can identify morphologic changes in the median nerve associated with CTS [37]. This includes median nerve enlargement at the level of the pisiform, flattening or notching of the nerve in the distal carpal tunnel and decreased nerve gliding with finger movements [38-40]. US can detect structural causes of CTS such as synovitis, ganglia, or muscular and vascular abnormalities. Combining US imaging with a minimally invasive device allows for visualization of key structures in the carpal tunnel without an open incision. The anatomic resolution capabilities of US are currently excellent (on the order of 100 UM) and will only continue to improve. US is also attractive because it is portable, rapid, and cost effective [41, 42-44].

US can define tunnel anatomy prior to surgery and identify high division of the median nerve where patients whose anatomy is not amenable to minimal access surgery. Nakamichi used US to measure the distance between the median nerve and ulnar neurovascular bundle in 60 wrists in 54 patients with surgically indicated idiopathic carpal tunnel. Patients with a measurement of <3 mm were treated with open surgery [45]. We agree and converted to open surgery in 2 of our patients. Chern performed a cadaver study using US to measure safety zones. The distance between the radial edge of the hook of the hamate to the median nerve was 4-8 mm with a mean of 5. The distance between the distal transverse carpal ligament and superficial palmar arch ranged from 6-16 mm with a median of 11 [46]. These studies support the safe and practical use of US in minimally invasive CTR [23, 41, 47], and prompted us to use US to identify the transverse carpal ligament, safe zones and median nerve during surgery in the featured minimally invasive cases with the MANOS CTR device.

The limitation of US is that it is operator dependent and has a learning curve with regard to transducer handling, obtaining high quality images and interpreting them, and accurately placing and visualizing instruments within the US beam. Furthermore, acoustic shadows from the MANOS CTR blade can obscure landmarks. Based on the author's experience, educational course in US is recommended if not routinely used in the physician's practice. US provides an excellent view of the carpal tunnel and its contents, requires minimal capital costs and is widely available. MANOS may be ideally suited for US-guided CTR due to its small device diameter and ability to introduce it into the carpal tunnel in a blunt or safe configuration. The combination of US, nerve stimulation and a minimally invasive cupping device proved to be a useful combination in minimizing surgical trauma and potentially improving patient recovery time. A larger prospective study is under way to further evaluate the safety and efficacy of the described technique.

MANOS carpal tunnel release results in quicker healing and return to activities of daily living comparable to endoscopic techniques. Three month functional severity and symptom severity scores compare favorably to endoscopic literature controls and are better than scores reported with open carpal tunnel release. In this study, average return to work was 14 days and in 18 days in the patients with occupational claims. Trumble reported an average return to work time of 18 days in 97 patients treated with endoscopic carpal tunnel release. Chow et al. reported in a retrospective study of endoscopic CT surgery in 456 patients that 59% returned to work in 2 weeks and 84% after 4 weeks [48]. Whereas, Masear et al. reported an average of 54 days of work loss after open carpal tunnel release [49].

One year follow-up of 89 patients treated with MANOS with a validated questionnaire are the same as open surgery. Standardized questionnaires are more sensitive to critical changes from carpal tunnel syndrome than physical measures [50]. Ninety three percent of our patients had good results at a year. There was one case of new first finger numbness and pain unresponsive to revision surgery and five other poor results for pain relief not treated with additional surgery. One other patient had incomplete release and had a good result with open release.

To date the author's experience is over a hundred cases and there have been a total of 2000 MANOS procedures performed. Adoption of new carpal tunnel technology is suppressed by several factors. The MANOS device adds cost to care of CTS when a cheap alternative exists i.e. open surgery with a scalpel. Other surgeons have limited experience with ultrasound and are not comfortable using this as the primary visualization modality for surgery. The majority want a large prospective randomized trial proving results are better before changing their practice patterns. Others argued that poor CTS results are due to overtreatment when indications are equivocal, lack of clarity of diagnosis and not the skin incision.

The MANOS CTR devise for minimally invasive carpal tunnel release results in quicker healing and return to activities of daily living and work at three months compared to open techniques. Three month results are comparable to endoscopic literature controls as accessed on validated outcome questionnaires. Definitive healing at one year is the same as with open and endoscopic surgery. Ultrasound has supplanted nerve stimulation method as the primary tool for surgical navigation and confirmation of ligament release.

References

[1]   Agee JM, Peimer CA, Pyrek JD, Walsh WE. Endoscopic carpal tunnel release: A prospective study of complications and surgical experience. *J Hand Surg Am* 1995;20: 165-172.

[2]   Boniface SJ, Morris I, Macleod A. How does neurophysiological assessment influence the management and outcome of patients with carpal tunnel syndrome? *J Rheumatology Br* 1994;33: 1169-1170.

[3]   Cresswell TR, Heras-Palou C, Bradley MJ, Chamberlain ST, Hartley RH, Dias JJ, Burke FD. Long-term outcome after carpal tunnel decompression - a prospective randomised study of the indiana tome and a standard limited palmar incision. *J Hand Surg Eur Vol* 2008;33: 332-336.

[4]   Hansen TB, Dalsgaard J, Meldgaard A, Larsen K. A prospective study of prognostic factors for duration of sick leave after endoscopic carpal tunnel release. *BMC Musculoskelet Disord* 2009;10: 144.

[5]   Pomerance J, Zurakowski D, Fine I. The cost-effectiveness of nonsurgical versus surgical treatment for carpal tunnel syndrome. *J Hand Surg Am* 2009;34: 1193-1200.

[6]   Williams AM, Baker PA, Platt AJ. The impact of dressings on recovery from carpal tunnel decompression. *J Plast Reconstr Aesthet Surg* 2008;61: 1493-1495.

[7]   Cellocco P, Rossi C, Bizzarri F, Patrizio L, Costanzo G. Mini-open blind procedure versus limited open technique for carpal tunnel release: A 30-month follow-up study. *J Hand Surg Am* 2005;30: 493-499.

[8]   Katz JN, Larson MG, Fossel AH, Liang MH. Validation of a surveillance case definition of carpal tunnel syndrome. *J Public Health Am* 1991;81: 189-193.

[9]   Lewicky RT. Endoscopic carpal tunnel release: The guide tube technique. *Arthroscopy* 1994;10: 39-49.

[10]   Siegmeth AW, Hopkinson-Woolley JA. Standard open decompression in carpal tunnel syndrome compared with a modified open technique preserving the superficial skin nerves: A prospective randomized study. *J Hand Surg* 2006;31A: 1483-1489.

[11]   Wilson KM. Double incision open technique for carpal tunnel release: An alternative to endoscopic release. *J Hand Surg* 1994;19A: 907-912.

[12]   Agee JM, McCaroll HR, Tortosa RD, Berry DA, Szabo RM, Peimer CA. Endoscopic release of the carpal tunnel: A randomized prospective multicenter study. *J Hand Surg* 1992;17A:987-995.

[13]   Brown RA, Gelberman RH, Seiler JG, Abrahamsson SO, Weiland AJ, Urbaniak JR et al. Carpal tunnel release. A prospective, randomized assessment of open and endoscopic methods. *J Bone Joint Surg* 1993;75A:1265-1275.

[14]   Kerr CD, Gittins ME, Sybert DR. Endoscopic versus open carpal tunnel release: clinical results. *Arthroscopy* 1994;10:266-269.

[15]   Hamed AR, Makki D, Chari R, Packer G. Double-versus single-incision technique for open carpal tunnel release. *Orthopedics* 2009;32:733.

[16]   Boeckstyns ME, Sorensen AI. Does endoscopic carpal tunnel release have a higher rate of complications than open carpal tunnel release? An analysis of published series. *J Hand Surg* 1999;24B:9-15.

[17]   Cellocco P, Rossi C, El Boustany S, Di Tanna GL, Costanzo G. Minimally invasive carpal tunnel release. *Orthop Clin North Am* 2009;40:441-448.

[18]   Zyluk A, Strychar J. A comparison of two limited open techniques for carpal tunnel release. *J Hand Surg* 2006;31B:466-472.

[19]   Tan T, Yeo C, Smith E. High definition ultrasound as diagnostic adjunct for incomplete carpal tunnel release. *Hand Surg* 2011;16: 289.

[20]   Bodor M, Lesher JM, Colio S. Ultrasound guided hand, wrist, and elbow injections. SN Narouze. *Atlas of ultrasound-guided procedures in interventional pain management.* New York: Springer; 2011:307-321.

[21]   Macaire P, Singelyn F, Narchi P, Paqueron X. Ultrasound- or nerve stimulation-guided wrist blocks for carpal tunnel release: A randomized prospective comparative study. *Reg Anes Pain Med* 2008;33: 363-368.

[22]   Nakamichi K, Tachibana S. Ultrasonographically assisted carpal tunnel release. *J Hand Surg* 1997;22A: 853-862.

[23]   Nakamichi K, Tachibana S, Yamamoto S, Ida M. Percutaneous carpal tunnel release compared with mini-open release using ultrasonographic guidance for both techniques. *J Hand Surg* 2010;35A: 437-445.

[24] Levine DW, Simmons BP, Koris MJ, Daltrov LH, Hohl GG, Fossel AH et al. A self-administered questionnaire for the assessment of severity of symptoms and functional status in carpal tunnel syndrome. *J Bone Joint Surg* 1993;75A:1585-1592.

[25] Nancollas MP, Peimer CA, Wheeler DR, Sherwin FS. Long-term results of carpal tunnel release. *J Hand Surg* 1995;20B:470-474.

[26] Vasiliadis HS, Xenakis TA, Mitsionis G, Paschos N, Georgoulis A. Endoscopic versus open carpal tunnel release. *Arthroscopy* 2010;26:26-33.

[27] Ferrari GP, Gilbert A. The superficial anastomosis on the palm of the hand between the ulnar and median nerves. *J Hand Surg* 1991;16B:511-514.

[28] Meals RA, Shaner M. Variations in digital sensory patterns: a study of the ulnar nerve-median nerve palmar communicating branch. *J Hand Surg* 1983;8A:411-414.

[29] May JW, Rosen H. Division of the Sensory Ramus Communicans between the Ulnar and Median Nerves: A Complication Following Carpal Tunnel Release. *J Bone Joint Surg* 1981;63A:836-838.

[30] Arner M, Hagberg L, Rosen B. Sensory disturbances after two-portal endoscopic carpal tunnel release: a preliminary report. *J Hand Surg* 1994;19A:548-551.

[31] McCormack B, Bowen W, Gunther S, Linthicum J, Kaplan M, Eyster E. Carpal tunnel release using the MANOS CTR system: Preliminary results in 52 patients. *J Hand Surg Am* 2012;37-689-694.

[32] Kirkpatrick PJ, Watters G, Strong AJ, Walliker JR, Gleeson MJ. Prediction of facial nerve function after surgery for cerebellopontine angle tumors: use of a facial nerve stimulator and monitor. *Skull Base Surg* 1991;1:171-176.

[33] Lamphier TA. A nerve stimulator providing easy identification of the facial nerve and its branches. *Am J Surg* 1954;88:674-676.

[34] Page C, Peltier J, Charlet L, Laude M, Strunski V. Superior approach to the inferior laryngeal nerve in thyroid surgery: anatomy, surgical technique and indications. *Surg Radiol Anat* 2006;28:631-636.

[35] Prithvi Raj P, Rosenblatt R, Montgomery SJ. Use of the nerve stimulator for peripheral blocks. *J Reg Anesth Pain Med* 1980;5:14-21.

[36] Ford DJ, Pither C, Raj PP. Comparison of insulated and uninsulated needles for locating peripheral nerves with a peripheral nerve stimulator. *Anesth Analg* 1984;63:925-928.

[37] Kamolz LP, Schrogendorger KF, Rab M, Girsch W, Gruber H, Frey M. The precision of ultrasound imaging and its relevance for carpal tunnel syndrome. *Surg Radiol Anat* 2000;23: 117-121.

[38] French C, Cartwright MS, Hobson-Webb LD, Boon AJ, Alter KE, Hunt CH, Flores VH, Werner RA, Shook SJ, Thomas TD, Primack SJ, Walker FO. Evidence-based guideline: Neuromuscular ultrasound for the diagnosis of carpal tunnel syndrome. *Muscle Nerve* 2012;46: 287-293.

[39] Ashraf AR, Jali R, Moghtaderi AR, Yazdani AH. The diagnostic value of ultrasonography in patients with electrophysiologicaly confirmed carpal tunnel syndrome. *Elect Clin Neuro* 2009;49: 3-8.

[40] Lee DL, van Holsbeeck MT, Janevski PK, Ganos DL, Ditmars DM, Darian VB. Diagnosis of carpal tunnel syndrome: Ultrasound versus electromyography. *Rad Clin N Am* 1999;37: 859-872.

[41] Lecoq B, Hanouz N, Vielpeau C, Marcelli C. Ultrasound-guided percutaneous surgery for carpal tunnel syndrome: A cadaver study. *Joint Bone Spine* 2011;78: 516-518.

[42] Abicalaf CA, de Barros N, Sernik RA, Pimentel BF, Braga-Baiak A, Braga L, Houvet P, Brasseur JL, Roger B, Cerri GG. Ultrasound evaluation of patients with carpal tunnel syndrome before and after endoscopic release of the transverse carpal ligament. *Clin Radiol* 2007;62: 891-896.

[43] Ettema AM, Belohlavek M, Zhao C, Oh SH, Amadio PC, An KN. High-resolution ultrasound analysis of subsynovial connective tissue in human cadaver carpal tunnel. *J Orthop Res* 2006;24: 2011-2020.

[44] Yoshii Y, Villarraga HR, Henderson J, Zhao C, An KN, Amadio PC. Ultrasound assessment of the displacement and deformation of the median nerve in the human carpal tunnel with active finger motion. *J Bone Joint Surg Am* 2009;91: 2922-2930.

[45] Nakamichi K, Tachibana S. Distance between the median nerve and ulnar neurovascular bundle: Clinical significance with ultrasonographically assisted carpal tunnel release. *J Hand Surg* 1998;23A: 870-874.

[46] Chern TC, Jou IM, Chen WC, Wu KC, Shao CJ, Shen PC. An ultrasonographic and anatomical study of carpal tunnel, with special emphasis on the safe zones in percutaneous release. *J Hand Surg Eur Vol* 2009;34: 66-71.

[47] Rowe NM, Michaels J, Soltanian H, Dobryansky M, Peimer CA, Gurtner GC. Sonographically guided percutaneous carpal tunnel release. *Ann Plast Surg* 2005;55: 52-56.

[48] Chow, JC. The Chow technique of endoscopic release of the carpal
      ligament for carpal tunnel syndrome: four years of clinical results.
      Arthroscopy 1993;9:301-314.
[49] Masear VR, Hayes JM, Hyde AG. An industrial cause of carpal tunnel
      syndrome. *J Hand Surg Am.* 1986;11:222-227.
[50] Amadio PC, Silverstein MD, Ilstrup DM, Schleck CD, Jensen LM.
      Outcome   assessment   for   carpal   tunnel   surgery: the   relative
      responsiveness of generic, arthritis-specific, disease-specific, and
      physical examination measures. *J Hand Surg* 1996;21A:338-346.

In: Carpal Tunnel Syndrome
Editor: Morton Ledford

ISBN: 978-1-63321-142-1
© 2014 Nova Science Publishers, Inc.

Chapter 3

Quantification of Behavioral Consequences of Carpal Tunnel Syndrome: Insights from Biomechanical Analysis of Grasping and Manipulation

Wei Zhang[1]* and Marco Santello[2]
[1]Department of Physical Therapy, College of Staten Island,
City University of New York, Staten Island, NY, US
[2]School of Biological and Health Systems Engineering,
Arizona State University, Tempe, AZ, US

Abstract

Carpal Tunnel Syndrome (CTS) is known to affect manual dexterity. Electrodiagnostic tests are often used to quantify the extent of damage (mild to severe) of the median nerve. However, these clinical measures of median nerve damage cannot be used to quantify the extent of hand functional deficits. To address this question, several recent studies have been conducted to quantify the behavioral effects of CTS on patients'

---

* Corresponding author: Wei Zhang, Department of Physical Therapy, 2800 Victory Blvd, Building 5N – 207, College of Staten Island/City University of New York, Staten Island, NY 10314, USA, Ph.: +1-718-982-2989, Fax: +1-718-982-2984, E-mail: wei.zhang@ csi.cuny.edu.

ability to perform grasping and dexterous manipulation. These studies have used biomechanical analyses to identify functional deficits in hand control due to sub-optimal sensorimotor integration caused by reduced tactile sensitivity at a subset of the digits. We review published studies and present novel findings about the effects of CTS on patients' sensorimotor deficits. These deficits are revealed by tasks that require the ability to integrate sensory feedback with motor commands for coordinating digit forces and position. The findings of this research have shown that chronic median nerve compression affects the ability to coordinate preprogrammed and feedback-driven control for effective and efficient force adaptation in multi-digit grasping.

Introduction

The hand is essential to human motor behavior and is one of the most studied and complex motor systems. Its elaborate biomechanical and neural architecture underlies its ability to assume a uniquely rich repertoire of postures that can mold and exert forces onto virtually any object, enabling us to perform an incredible range of manipulatory behaviors. For successful object manipulation, somatosensory feedback (from tactile, joint and muscle receptors) about object properties must be integrated with motor commands, i.e., sensorimotor integration. For example, when lifting a glass, properties such as center of mass, weight, and texture need to be accurately sensed by the hand to select an appropriate distribution of digit forces such that the glass neither slips or tilts, nor crushes. Effective control of digit forces relies on both anticipatory and feedback-driven control mechanisms, each of which requires sensorimotor integration.

The ability to anticipate object properties is based on acquiring, storing and retrieving memories associated with previous manipulations of a given object (Gordon et al., 1993, Jenmalm et al., 1997; Johansson, 1998; Johansson and Westling, 1984, 1987, 1988a, b; Salimi et al., 2000, 2003). This mechanism is used to plan and execute – in an anticipatory fashion – the forces necessary to manipulate an object without having to rely on sensing object properties that would occur during object manipulation, e.g., before the object is lifted (Fu et al., 2010; Zhang et al., 2010). Feedback mechanisms are known to play a crucial role in upgrading erroneously planned fingertip forces (Augurelle et al., 2003; Johansson, 1996, 1998; Macefield, 1996; Monzee et al., 2003; for review see Johansson and Flanagan 2009). In healthy subjects, the coordination of digit forces has been extensively studied across the different phases of grasping, e.g., force rise (i.e., from contact with the object to onset of object manipulation), object manipulation (i.e., lift), static hold, or dynamic transport of the object, and object release (Forssberg et al., 1991, 1992; Rearick et al., 2002, 2003; Rearick and Santello, 2002; Reilmann et al., 2001; Santello and Soechting, 2000; Smith and Soechting, 2005). The force rise phase is important to assess anticipatory force mechanisms, whereas lift and hold phases are important to detect changes in digit force coordination that might be elicited by feedback mechanisms.

Studies in healthy individuals have suggested that visual and somatosensory feedback need to be processed and integrated with motor commands such as to initiate the complex spatial and temporal coordination of the digits required for skilled manipulatory behaviors (Gordon et al., 1993; Jenmalm and Johansson, 1997; Jenmalm et al., 2000; Johansson and Cole, 1994; Salimi et al., 2003). However, the delicate multi-digit force coordination that can be flexibly adapted to object properties (such as size, friction and weight) can be disrupted by a number of neurological and musculoskeletal diseases, such as Carpal Tunnel Syndrome (CTS). CTS is a compression neuropathy of the median nerve resulting in 1) somatosensory deficits in the thumb, index, middle and lateral half of the ring finger, and, in severe cases, 2) motor deficits in the thumb. Prolonged mechanical compression of the nerve can result in ischemic damage and/or changes in the myelination of the nerve, which in turn leads to slowing of axonal conduction velocity, nerve block, and in severe cases axonal loss (Nora et al., 2004; Welford, 1972). Patients with CTS suffer from a constellation of symptoms including aching and burning, tingling, numbness, weakness and clumsiness in the affected hand. In addition, CTS is one of the most common neuromuscular diseases affecting hand function and therefore dexterous manual tasks performed during activities of daily living. Physicians often hear complains such as 'easily dropping objects', or 'having problems with buttoning the shirt' from patients who have been diagnosed as CTS. It affects 6 to 14 million adults in the United States and there is a 10% lifetime risk of developing the syndrome. Complications from CTS result in an average of 25 days lost from work per employee per year (Wing, 2006) with an average lifetime cost of $30,000 per individual in the U.S. (fact sheet by NINDS). It is estimated that 400,000 CTS surgeries are performed in the US each year (Mondelli et al. 2004). Because of the high prevalence of this disorder and its potential for disability, it is imperative that effective techniques quantifying complex aspects of grasping and manipulatory behaviors be made available to clinicians to help improve diagnosis and determine the effectiveness of clinical interventions. While the physiological and pathological perspectives of CTS has been extensively studied and established, especially in available diagnosis methodology and treatment assessment (see review Jablecki et al., 1993; Massy-Westropp et. al., 2000; Verdugo et al., 2008), much less is known about the effect of CTS on sensorimotor integration underlying the control of grasping and manipulation.

Additionally, we start to appreciate the fundamental significance of sensorimotor integration on manipulatory behavior when the use of somatosensory information from the digits is impaired by a neuropathy or neurological disorder. Associated with somatosensory deficits in the thumb, index, middle and lateral half of the ring fingers, CTS poses unique challenges for the Central Nervous System (CNS) for whole-hand manipulation as it selectively impairs sensorimotor function at a subset of digits. This raises the question of how the CNS integrates sensory information, from CTS-affected and non-affected digits, with motor commands to fine-tune digit forces to task requirement. As such, CTS can be used as a model to provide insight into the mechanisms of mapping "noisy" somatosensory feedback into motor commands for anticipatory and reactive force control responsible for skilled object manipulation. In this, we review recent findings from our work based on biomechanical analysis of multi-digit force adaptation and coordination as a function of object properties and grip type.

CTS and Control of Object Grasping and Manipulation

It is believed that repetitive motion of the hand is a major factor of pathogenesis of cumulative trauma disorders (Kiser 1987). For example, the high prevalence of CTS is reported in occupations characterized by large and repetitive hand forces (Silverstein et al. 1987). It has been suggested that CTS maybe caused by the tendon and nerve movement during prolonged repetitive hand movement (Ugbolue et al. 2005), as well as the migration of lumbrical muscles into the carpal tunnel during fingers' active flexion movement, thus leading to increased carpal tunnel pressure (Siegel et al. 1995; Yii and Elliot 1994; Cobb et al. 1995). Driven by its high prevalence, CTS has been recognized in many recent studies in investigating biomechanical characteristics of carpal tunnel structures (Xiu et al. 2010), efficacy of conservative treatments or theoretical basis for surgical treatments in CTS patients (Li et al. 2009; Guo et al. 2009; Massy-Westropp et. al., 2000;

Verdugo et al., 2008). Despite studies that focused on the biomechanical, physiological, and pathological perspectives of CTS, there has been little research on the impact of CTS on activities of daily living. For an example, taking a sip from a glass requires a series of actions including objects' grasping and lifting while generating accurate forces and moment of force.

In a series of recent studies, we investigated the effects of CTS on sensorimotor integration revealed by the learning and adaptation of multi-digit coordination patterns during object grasping and manipulation (Zhang et al. 2011, 2012, 2013; Afifi et al. 2012).

These studies used the following protocol:

1) As one of the exclusion criteria, patients affected by severe CTS have been excluded from our studies as severe CTS affects thumb motor function. Therefore, only patients diagnosed with mild or moderate CTS severity, as well as age- and gender- matched controls, were recruited for our studies. This approach enabled us to focus on CTS-induced sensory deficits (please see Zhang et al. 2011 for a detailed description of inclusion and exclusion criteria).

2) The hand-held object to be manipulated was a customized inverted-T-shape grip device (**Figure** 1), attached with five six-component force/torque transducers (F/T, ATI Industrial Automation) to measure forces and moment-of-forces produced by each digit. A position/orientation sensor (P/O, Polhemus Fastrak) was positioned on the top of the object to determine the occurrence and magnitude of object roll during lift.

3) We instructed subjects 'to grasp, lift, hold (~4 s) and replace the object while keeping its vertical orientation'.

4) We systematically altered object properties to investigate multi-digit force coordination and adaptation. Our studies focused on the modulation of digit forces to object mass (Zhang et al. 2011, 2013), mass distribution (Zhang et al. 2012), and surface texture (Afifi et al. 2012). No explicit cues were given to subjects about these properties such that subjects had to sense (on a given trial) and recall (on subsequent trials) a given object property experienced on previous trial(s).

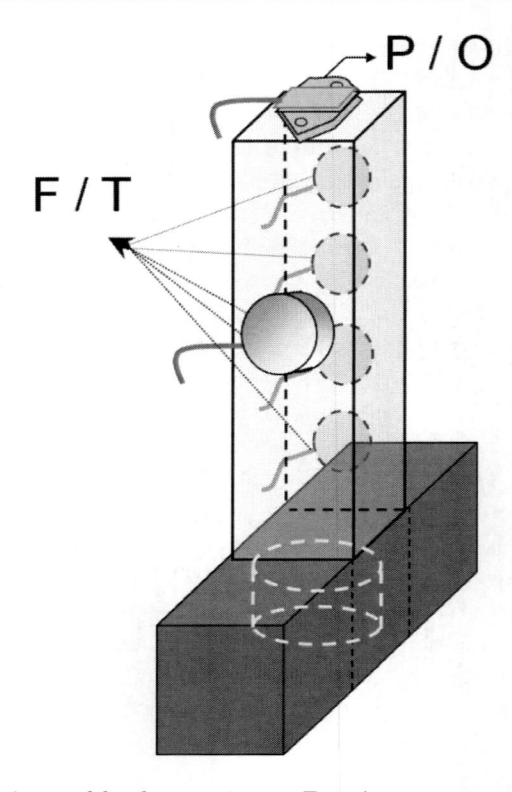

Figure 1. *Grip device used for the experiments.* Force/torque sensors (F/T) are mounted on both sides of the device to measure forces and moment of forces exerted by each digit (thumb, index, middle, ring, and little fingers: T, I, M, R, and L, respectively). A position/orientation (P/O) sensor was mounted on the top of the device to measure object kinematics. An extra mass could be inserted at the bottom of the grip device to alter experimental conditions in object weight (i.e., three weight conditions in Experiment 1: 445, 545, and 745 g; and two weight conditions in Experiment 4: light vs. heavy) or in object mass distribution (i.e., three center of mass conditions in Experiment 2: mass on the thumb, center, or finger sides; T_{CM}, C_{CM} and F_{CM}, respectively). Additionally, F/T sensors' surface could be covered with different textures when altering object texture experimental conditions (i.e., two texture conditions in Experiment 3: silk vs. sandpaper). The figure is from Wei Zhang et al. 2011 with authors' permission.

Mechanically, grasping and lifting an object while maintaining its vertical orientation (in 2-dimentional space) can be decomposed into two sub-tasks: 1) translate an object vertically against gravity; and 2) achieve equilibrium of resultant moment of force applied on the object. For the *vertical object translation sub-task*, prevention of object slip or drop requires the total tangential forces (also referred to as "load force", which is exerted parallel to the object surface) exerted by all of the involved digits to be larger (e.g., during object lift) or equal (e.g., during object hold) to the object weight. Consequently, the total normal force (also referred to as "grip force", which is exerted orthogonal to the object surface) should be sufficiently large so that the normal-to-tangential force ratio at each digit is greater than the ratio at which slip would occur (safety margin; Westling and Johansson 1984). Additionally, the normal force exerted by the thumb and the opposing digit(s) must be equal in magnitude, and opposite in direction, to avoid horizontal translation. For the *moment equilibrium sub-task*, the resultant moments exerted on the object in the frontal plane must be equal to zero. In this scenario, moments exerted by all of the involved digits must be either equivalent to zero when lifting an object with symmetric mass distribution, or non-zero to counterbalance an external moment caused, for example, by the object's asymmetrical mass distribution. Although the above mechanical requirements constrain how digit forces must be coordinated, there are other digit force parameters that are not constrained by the task mechanics. For example, maximal grip force is not uniquely defined by the task - as long as the object is not fragile, even though there is a requirement of minimum grip force required by the need to prevent object slip. Additionally, normal force sharing patterns among individual fingers are not defined by the task, i.e., subjects can still satisfy the above-described mechanical requirements while adopting many different multi-digit force sharing patterns.

CTS and Anticipatory Grasp Control

In healthy individuals, to successfully accomplish above task requirement, visual and somatosensory feedback is processed and integrated with motor commands to control multiple digit forces (Gordon et al. 1993; Jenmalm and Johansson, 1997; Jenmalm et al. 2000; Johansson and Cole, 1994; Salimi et al. 2003). Task-specific sensorimotor memory of complex spatial and temporal coordination of the digits can be formed upon exposure to repetitive hand-object interactions, and retrieved before grasp execution on subsequent trials. Experimentally, sensorimotor learning has been examined by quantifying how multi-digit force coordination patterns are flexibly adapted to object properties such as weight (Gordon et al. 1993), mass distribution (Fu et al., 2010), and friction (Aoki et al. 2006) in an anticipatory fashion (i.e., before object lift onset). These findings raise two questions regarding the extent to which CTS patients, affected by impaired sensation at a subset of the digits, can accurately perform grasp and manipulation: Would CTS patients be able to implement anticipatory grasp control to adapt multi-digit forces to object properties? If so, would they be able to use the same control strategies as healthy controls?

The results of our recent studies indicate that CTS patients were able to grasp, lift, hold, and replace objects as instructed. Furthermore, CTS patients could still learn to adapt multi-digit forces to different object properties as quickly as healthy controls. Specifically, after experiencing manipulation of same object for 1 to 2 trials, CTS patients started to modulate multi-digit forces as a function of object weight, mass distributions, and textures in an anticipatory fashion. This ability of CTS patients to implement anticipatory digit force control was revealed by a series of experiments (Experiments 1, 2, 3 and 4).

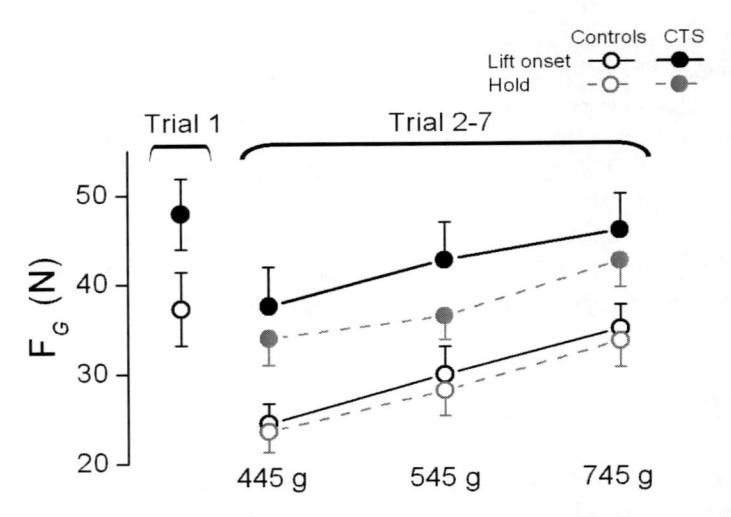

Figure 2. *Grip force at object lift onset and object hold.* Grip force (F_G) at object lift onset and during object hold on the 1st trial (averaged across all weights), and averaged across trials 2 through 7 are shown for the CTS and control groups (filled and open symbols, respectively) and each weight condition. Note that F_G during object hold on the first trial is not plotted since F_G did not change significantly across trials, i.e., F_G during hold on the first trial = F_G on trials 2-7. Vertical error bars denote standard errors. The figure is from Wei Zhang et al. 2011 with authors' permission.

In Experiment 1 (Zhang et al., 2011), both CTS and healthy controls were asked to grasp and lift an object with different weights. Note that changing object's mass affects the object vertical translation sub-task only, but not the moment equilibrium sub-task (see above). Similarly to healthy controls, CTS patients learned to scale multi-digit forces to object weight at object lift onset, as shown by larger grip force (Figure 2) and rate of grip force development for heavier objects without causing object roll. Similar CTS patients' ability of anticipatory force control to object weight was also observed in a later experiment (Experiment 4), which further revealed that CTS patients' anticipatory scaling of digit force was not affected by switching grip types requiring using a different number of digits to perform the same grasp and manipulation task (Zhang et al. 2013). In Experiment 2 (Zhang et al., 2012), object mass was the same across trials, but mass distribution was changed across blocks of consecutive trials to quantify the extent to which CTS patients could perform the moment of force sub-task. Using an object with an asymmetrical mass distribution resulted in object roll during lift on the first couple of trials. Nevertheless, object roll was minimized on subsequent trials to ~2 degrees. This is again evidence of accurate anticipatory control of a compensatory moment before the object was lifted off the table.

These findings suggest that CTS patients maintain a residual ability to process sensory feedback, form sensorimotor memories, retrieve and use them to modulate multi-digit forces prior to object lift onset. Given the sensory deficits identified by electrodiagnostic tests (details see Zhang et al. 2011), possible explanations for this residual ability to modulate digital force to object weight and mass distribution are that spared somatosensory feedback from the hand and/or that more proximal sources of feedback (such as proprioception feedback) were also utilized. Specifically, it is possible that sensory feedback from muscle, joint, and tendon mechanoreceptors in the forearm and upper arm (whose function is spared by median nerve compression) could have been integrated with residual somatosensory feedback from the hand to infer object weight and mass distribution, and coordinate digit forces after the first couple of object lifts.

Similarly, when grip surface texture was changed across blocks of trials (Experiment 3; Afifi et al. 2012), CTS patients could learn to modulate digit forces to frictional properties (slippery vs. rough) of the grasped surface. Unlike the above interpretation of the results from the studies of object mass or mass distribution, it is unlikely that spared muscle, joint, and tendon mechanoreceptors in the forearm and upper arm played a significant role in force adaptation to texture. This is because such modulation is generally attributed to tactile mechanoreceptors in the fingertips (Birznieks et al. 2001; for review see Johansson and Flanagan 2009). We suggest the successful force adaptation to texture exhibited by CTS patients indicate the existence of spared tactile afferent fibers from the CTS-affected digits and/or the integration of afferent input acquired through the non-affected digits (i.e., little and ulnar half of the ring finger) to discriminate different textures. Additional analyses revealed that CTS patients might have increased their digit contact time to allow for tactile information to be sensed and processed given the slowing in their sensory nerve conduction.

CTS and Deficits in Sensorimotor Learning

Our findings suggest that, although CTS did not significantly affect patients' ability to perform object grasp and manipulation tasks, it interfered with the modulation of specific grasp control variables denoting CTS-induced deficits in the sensorimotor integration process. Specifically, CTS patients showed a reduced ability relative to controls to use prior experience in modulating multi-digit forces in an anticipatory fashion, i.e., at object lift onset. In fact, grip force modulation by CTS patients did not discriminate across weights and centers of mass as accurately as controls. Patients' lower discrimination was observed between light object weights in parallel with larger across-trial variability in digit force control (Experiment 1; Zhang et al., 2011), and between center and off-center mass distributions (Experiment 2; Zhang et al., 2012). Both findings underscore the importance of tactile feedback on fine regulation and reproducibility of digit force modulation to object properties.

Another deficit in anticipatory control was the CTS patients' reduced ability to balance digit forces, resulting in unnecessary net moments at object lift onset when lifting objects with a symmetrical center of mass (Zhang et al., 2011). In contrast, CTS patients learned to plan a compensatory moment to minimize object roll to the same extent as controls when lifting objects with asymmetrical mass distribution (Zhang et al., 2012). It should be noted that the discrepancy in CTS patients' difficulty in maintaining a zero moment versus their ability in anticipating a non-zero moment does not imply that CTS affects force adaptation to object mass to a greater extent than adaptation to object center of mass. As a matter of fact, in the latter scenario, multi-digit force coordination in controls fully exploited the available degrees of freedom that contribute to compensatory moment generation: modulation of digit normal forces, tangential forces, and the location of the net center of pressure on the finger side of the device at object lift onset (Figure 3). In contrast, patients modulated *only* the finger net center pressure at object lift onset by modulating normal force sharing patterns while using the same normal and tangential forces across all object mass distribution conditions. This finding can be interpreted as solving the problem of redundant degrees of freedom by 'freezing' a subset of degrees of freedom (Bernstein, 1967; Newell, 1991; Vereijken et al. 1992). The use of this strategy might have been preferable because the modulation of one variable while keeping two other variables constant might be easier to implement than concurrent modulation of three variables as found in controls. This phenomenon might be indicative of a lower degree of flexibility of the sensorimotor system in CTS to adapt to grasp task conditions. The selective modulation of the net center of pressure also indicates that residual tactile and proprioceptive feedback in CTS can be more effectively integrated with motor commands for generating individuated finger forces than for the fine scaling of finger force magnitude. This might account for patients' reliance on exploiting finger force sharing pattern modulation to attain the desired compensatory moment.

Moreover, when the object to be manipulated was of same weight and mass distribution but different textures (Afifi et al. 2012), healthy controls tended to use a "probing" strategy prior to lifting the object by continually modulating their digit normal forces between contact and object lift-off. This suggests the healthy controls actively used sensory feedback to fine-tune their digit forces. However, this probing strategy was not evident in CTS patients, suggesting either (1) an inability to use sensory feedback to finely regulate forces, or (2) a compensatory strategy chosen by the CTS patients, i.e., the use of excessive forces, which nevertheless would preclude fine regulation of digit forces. These findings suggest that, although CTS did not affect patients' ability to perform object grasp and manipulation task, it interfered with the modulation of specific grasp control variables.

In conclusion, CTS patients exhibited deficits in sensorimotor integration as revealed by higher across-trial digit force variability, reduced ability to use prior experience to scale digit forces, lower discrimination of force modulation to lighter object weights or to center of mass, and a lower ability to minimize net moments on the object at lift onset. These findings indicate that CTS significantly affects the quality of grasp control. Therefore, we conclude that CTS does not affect macroscopic features of grasp control when adapting multi-digit forces to object properties. Nevertheless, chronic median nerve compression affects the ability to coordinate preprogrammed and feedback-driven control for effective and efficient grip force adaptation thus denoting deficits in sensorimotor integration. The above-described behavioral deficits, although relatively subtle, result from patients' reduced ability to generate, store, and retrieve accurate sensorimotor memories of previous manipulations, thus preventing them from fully compensating for impaired somatosensory feedback. Therefore, CTS patients do not benefit from consecutive practice with object manipulation. This phenomenon leads to the inability to plan and execute manipulation as efficiently as controls.

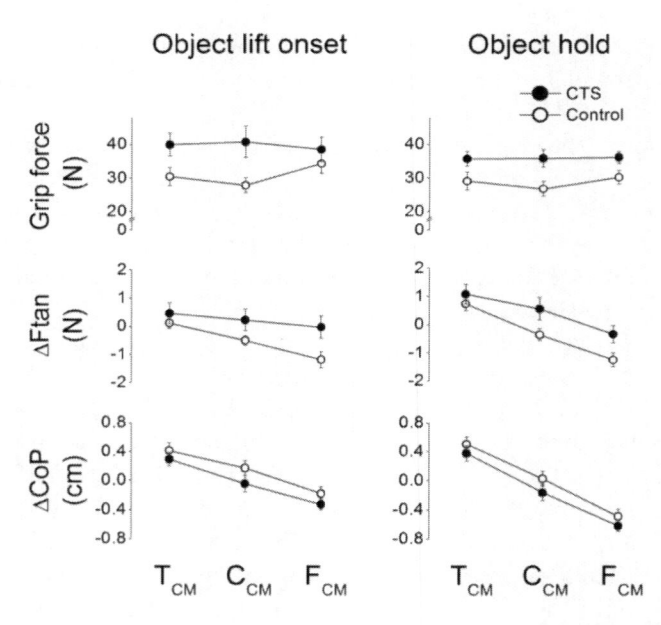

Figure 3. *Compensatory moment components*. Grip force (F_G), the difference between thumb and finger tangential forces (ΔFtan), and the vertical distance between thumb and finger center of pressure applied on each side of the grip device (ΔCoP) at object lift onset and hold (left and right column, respectively). Data are mean values averaged across trial 4 through 7 for each subject group and mass distribution condition. Vertical bars denote standard errors. The figure is from Wei Zhang et al. 2012 with authors' permission.

CTS and Excessive Grip Force

In our studies of whole-hand grasping (i.e., five digits), we have consistently found that CTS patients tend to exert significantly larger digit normal forces than controls, irrespective of the grasping task requirement of multi-digit force modulation to object weight, mass distribution, or texture. Specifically, while exhibiting abilities to effectively scale grip force to object properties and develop multi-digit forces and compensatory moment, CTS patients' task performance was inefficient as they consistently exerted excessive forces on the object when compared to controls. This excessive force compared to controls was observed very early in the grasp on the first lifting trial, from object lift onset to object hold, and regardless of object properties, suggesting the use of a possible preprogrammed control mechanism. These observations indicate that CTS-induced sensorimotor deficits interfere with sensorimotor integration processes associated with anticipatory control mechanisms. Excessive grip force in CTS patients may represent an attempt to compensate for their sensorimotor dysfunction (slowing in sensory nerve conduction) by prioritizing effectiveness, i.e., preventing the object from slipping, over efficiency, i.e., producing just sufficient force for holding the object against gravity.

We should emphasize that CTS patients' tendency for exerting excessive grip forces does not necessarily imply a preprogrammed, 'default' strategy, as suggested by our recent CTS study on the effects of CTS on grasp control using a variable number of digits, i.e., thumb-index, thumb-index-middle, thumb-index-middle-ring, and all digits (Zhang et al. 2013). We found that the above tendency for exerting excessively large grip force in CTS patients was grip-type dependent. Specifically, CTS patients exerted excessive grip force but only for manipulations involving *both* CTS-affected and non-affected digits, i.e., thumb-index-middle-ring and thumb-index-middle-ring-little fingers (Figure 4). In contrast, patients and controls exerted similar grip force when using only CTS-affected digits. This finding is novel but counterintuitive, since patients exerted significantly larger normal forces when the more sensate digits, i.e., the ring finger, or the ring and little fingers, were added to the grasp (Figure 4). This was due to the CTS patients' producing significantly larger normal forces in the ring and little fingers than the controls, which were not sufficiently compensated for by the reduction of normal forces at the index and middle fingers. The fact that healthy controls used the same grip force across all grip types is evidence of efficient force coordination and control, and suggests that the intact CNS is not challenged by varying the number of digits in the grasp. The larger grip force exhibited by patients suggest that the effects of CTS on manipulation control are dependent on the number of digits engaged in the task, and more specifically that the combination of CTS-affected and non-affected digits leads to greater digit force coordination deficits than grips involving CTS-affected digits only. It is therefore conceivable that the process of integrating intact and reduced sensory feedback from the fingertips might be more challenging to CNS than integrating feedback from CTS-affected digits only. While our interpretation requires further investigation, experimental evidence suggests that chronic CTS results in changes within the somatosensory system that has the potential to affect the activity of the ulnar nerve-innervated ring and little fingers. Specifically, Tinazzi et al. (1998) observed increased sensory evoked potentials in the hand somatosensory cortex of CTS patients after stimulation of the ulnar nerve. How such changes in the sensory system with respect to ulnar nerve may affect the motor output of the ulnar nerve (i.e., ring and little finger) remains to be determined.

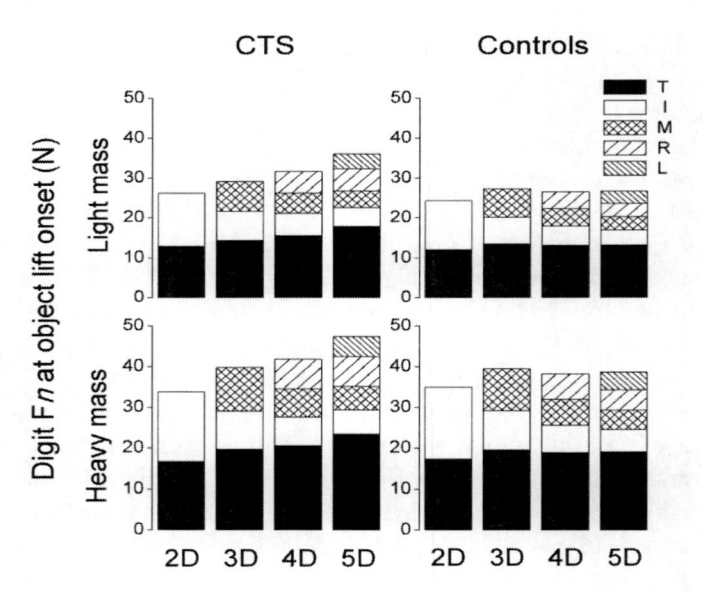

Figure 4. *Individual digit normal forces at object lift onset*. The normal force exerted by each digit at object lift onset is shown for each grip type, mass, and subject group (CTS and controls on the left and right column, respectively). Two-, three-, four- and five-digit grasps are denoted by 2D (Thumb-Index), 3D (Thumb-Index-Middle), 4D (Thumb-Index-Middle-Ring), and 5D (Thumb-Index-Middle-Ring-Little) respectively. Data are mean values averaged across trials 3 through 7 for each subject group. The figure is from Wei Zhang et al. 2013 with authors' permission.

CTS and Online Feedback Control

As described above, multi-digit force coordination quantified at object lift onset was used to examine anticipatory control mechanism responsible to object properties based on previous manipulations. Consequently, to evaluate subjects' ability of motor adaptation as a result of sensory feedback acquired following object lift onset, we have also quantified kinetic variables during the object hold phase. Following object lift and during object hold, sensory feedback about the manipulation (e.g., object tilt) becomes available through vision and residual somatosensory feedback, thus potentially allowing individuals to detect errors in the anticipatory control of grasp variables. Comparisons between these two temporal epochs should then allow the investigation of feedback-driven modulation of multi-digit forces.

One major finding based upon these comparisons was that healthy controls were able to anticipate grip force used to hold the object before lifting the object, whereas CTS patients further decreased grip force from object lift onset to object hold (Zhang et al., 2011). That is, unlike controls, CTS patients consistently overshot, from the second trial onwards across consecutive trials, grip force before lifting the object (Figure 2). We interpret the consistently larger grip force at object lift onset than during the static phase as a strategy learned during everyday activity to compensate for deficits in tactile feedback signaling distinct events of the manipulation, e.g., force development prior to object lift, the dynamic force modulation during object lift, and isometric force generation during object hold. In addition, CTS patients may prefer to use an extra safety margin of grip forces particularly during the dynamic phase, as evidenced by the fact that the younger CTS patients use a consistent safety margin, i.e., normal force above that necessary to hold the object across object textures, whereas healthy individuals modify their safety margin based on object texture (Experiment 3; Afifi et al., 2012). These results suggest that patients might have greater difficulty in anticipating the digit forces necessary to perform the task during the dynamic lifting phase than the static hold phase. Given the CTS patients' decreased ability to discriminate object weights and larger across-trial force variability, we propose that this systematic force overshoot at object lift onset vs. object hold represent a compensatory strategy that reflects different requirements and challenges to grasp stability associated with dynamic vs. static phases of manipulation.

Interestingly, we also found that CTS patients did not modulate tangential force to object center of mass at object lift onset, whereas they started to do so during object hold (Zhang et al. 2012) (Figure 3). As noted above, controls fully exploited all three available degrees of freedom to generate a compensatory moment, while patients anticipatorily modulated only the finger net center pressure at object lift onset. This suggests that the proposed 'freezing of degrees of freedom' strategy used at lift-off was deliberate, as opposed to being unavoidable. Specifically, CTS patients might be particularly more conservative before the dynamic phase of the task than during the static phase as we suggested in our earlier work (Zhang et al., 2011). This is because avoidance of object slip or roll during the first 100–150 ms of object lift relies on feedforward control of the compensatory moment. Following object lift, however, the predictive component of compensatory moment control can be replaced by online feedback control. In addition to somatosensory feedback from the hand and the arm, vision of object orientation might have contributed to the modulation of tangential forces.

Classification of CTS-Induced Sensorimotor Integration Deficits

Our findings have shown that mild and moderate severity CTS does not affect patients' ability to perform object grasp and manipulation tasks, but that it interfered with the modulation of specific biomechanical variables. We therefore examined the specific biomechanical variables that could best distinguish grasp performance in CTS patients vs. controls, as a step towards identifying variables that could potentially be used to detect early signs of CTS-induced sensorimotor deficits. We addressed this question by using exploratory stepwise discriminant analysis on data collected in Experiment 2. We found two groups of variables that could correctly classify CTS patients and controls at different time epochs of our task. Specifically, before the object was lifted, tangential force exerted by index (Ftan_I) for the off-centered mass distribution conditions (mass on the finger or thumb sides) could account for 43% of the total variation explained by the statistical model while misclassifying only 4 out of 28 subjects into the wrong group (3 CTS patients and 1 control subject) (Figure 5A). While the object was held in the air, a combination of tangential and normal forces of the ring finger (mass on the thumb and finger side, respectively) as well as resultant tangential force control variable (mass on the finger side) could account for 58% total variation with totally 4 misclassified cases (2 CTS patients and 2 control subjects) (Fig. 5B). Therefore, it is the magnitude and distribution of tangential forces occurring during the off-centered mass distribution conditions that appear to be the predominant behavioral difference in manipulation control between CTS and controls. Interestingly, both index and ring fingers are affected by CTS and have opposite mechanical actions by contributing to the production of pronation and supination moments, respectively, when manipulating our grip device due to their position relative to the thumb (Figure 1). According to the mechanical advantage principle, i.e., larger force production in the element(s) with longer lever arms in moment of force productions (Buchanan et al., 1989, Prilustsky 2000), finger normal force sharing at the index and little fingers were modulated the most to object center of mass. This phenomenon was likely due to the need of modulating the net center of pressure on the finger side of the grip device as a function of object mass distribution (Figure 3). However, normal forces by index and little fingers were not identified as discriminant variables for quantifying subjects' group membership. These results might be related to the differential sensorimotor impairment caused by CTS to intrinsic and extrinsic hand muscles, these muscles being primarily involved with tangential and normal force production, respectively.

Discriminant analysis was successful in identifying the digit force coordination features that best distinguished between the CTS patients and healthy controls. However, a larger number of patients across different grasp and manipulative tasks are needed to further define task-generalizable discriminant variables that best separate CTS patients from healthy individuals.

CTS Future Studies

Our recent series of CTS studies have provided insight into the grasp control mechanisms affected by the chronic compression median nerve neuropathy, carpel tunnel syndrome. The quantification of multi-digit kinetic control variables during dexterous manipulation tasks has improved our understanding of the crucial role of sensory feedback on sensorimotor integration processes responsible for anticipatory and reactive force control. We believe that this knowledge and a better understanding of CTS-induced deficits in grasping and manipulation can be beneficial towards prevention and/or treatment of CTS. Specifically, this work could have important implications for understanding the impact of repetitive hand activities in the workplace on CTS symptoms, assisting clinicians in early and accurate CTS diagnostics and assessing the effectiveness of clinical interventions.

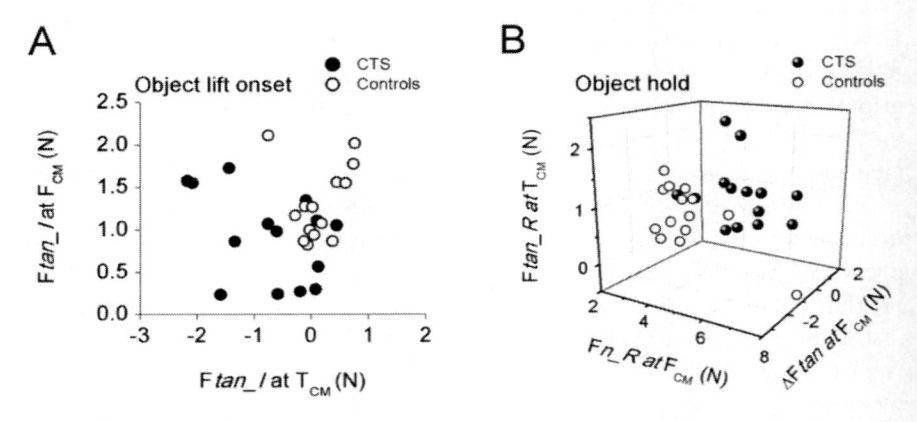

Figure 5. *Group classification based on stepwise discriminant analysis on digit forces at object lift onset and during object hold.* Statistically significant variables at object lift onset and during object hold (panels A and B, respectively) identified by stepwise discriminant analysis for differentiating CTS patients from controls. Panel A shows tangential force exerted by index finger when the mass was added on the finger or thumb side of the grip device (F_{CM} and T_{CM}, respectively) at object lift onset, whereas panel B shows tangential and normal force exerted by ring finger at T_{CM} and F_{CM}, respectively, together with the difference between thumb and finger tangential forces for the F_{CM} condition during object hold. Filled and open symbols denote data from CTS patients and controls.

References

Afifi, M; Santello, M; Johnston, J. A. Effects of carpal tunnel syndrome on adaptation of multi-digit forces to object texture. *Clinical Neurophysiology*, 2012, 123(11), 2281-2290.

Aoki, T; Niu, X; Latash, ML; Zatsiorsky, VM. Effects of friction at the digit-object interface on the digit forces in multi-finger prehension. *Exp Brain Res*, 2006, 172(4), 425-38.

Augurelle, AS; Smith, AM; Lejeune, T; Thonnard, JL. Importance of cutaneous feedback in maintaining a secure grip during manipulation of hand-held objects. *J Neurophysiol*, 2003, 89(2), 665-71.

Bernstein, NA: The co-ordination and regulation of movements. Oxford: Pergamon Press; 1967.

Birznieks, I; Jenmalm, P; Goodwin, AW; Johansson, RS. Encoding of direction of fingertip forces by human tactile afferents. *The Journal of Neuroscience*, 2001, 21(20), 8222-8237.

Brininger, TL; Rogers, JC; Holm, MB; Baker, NA; Li, ZM; Goitz, RJ. Efficacy of a fabricated customized splint and tendon and nerve gliding exercises for the treatment of carpal tunnel syndrome: a randomized controlled trial. *Archives of physical medicine and rehabilitation*, 2007, 88(11), 1429-1435.

Buchanan, TS; Rovai, GP; Rymer, WZ. Strategies for muscle activation during isometric torque generation at the human elbow. *J Neurophysiol*, 1989, 62, 1201–1212.

Buch-Jaeger, N; Foucher, G. Correlation of clinical signs with nerve conduction tests in the diagnosis of carpal tunnel syndrome. *J Hand Surg Br*, 1994, 19, 720–724.

Carpal tunnel syndrome fact sheet. National Institute of Neurological Disorders and Stroke; http://www.ninds.nih.gov/disorders/carpal_tunnel/detail_carpal_tunnel.htm.

Cobb, TK; An, KN; Cooney, WP. Effect of lumbrical muscle incursion within the carpal tunnel on carpal tunnel pressure: a cadaveric study. *J Hand Surg*, 1995; 20,186-92.

Cole, KJ; Steyers, CM; Graybill, EK. The effects of graded compression of the median nerve in the carpal canal on grip force. *Exp Brain Res*, 2003, 148, 150–157.

Flanagan, JR; King, S; Wolpert, DM; Johansson, RS. Sensorimotor prediction and memory in object manipulation. Can J Exp Psychol, 2001, 55, 89–97.

Forssberg, H; Eliasson, AC; Kinoshita, H; Johansson, RS; Westling, G. Development of human precision grip. I: Basic coordination of force. *Exp Brain Res*, 1991, 85, 451-57.

Forssberg, H; Kinoshita, H; Eliasson, AC; Johansson, RS; Westling, G; and, Gordon, AM. Development of human precision grip. II. Anticipatory control of isometric forces targeted for object's weight. *Exp Brain Res*, 1992, 90, 393-8.

Fu; Q, Zhang; W, Santello; M. Anticipatory planning and control of grasp positions and forces for dexterous two-digit manipulation. *The Journal of Neuroscience*, 2010, 30(27), 9117-9126.

Gordon, AM; Westling, G; Cole, KJ; Johansson, RJ. Memory representations underlying motor commands used during manipulation of common and novel objects. *J Neurophysiol*, 1993, 69, 1789-96.

Guo, X; Fan, Y; Li, ZM. Effects of dividing the transverse carpal ligament on the mechanical behavior of the carpal bones under axial compressive load: a finite element study. *Medical engineering & physics*, 2009, *31*(2), 188-194.

Hilburn, JW. General principles and use of electrodiagnostic studies in carpal and cubital tunnel syndromes. *Hand Clin*, 1996, 12, 205–221.

Jablecki; CK; Andary, CMT; So, YT; Wilkins, DE; Williams, FH; AAEM. Quality Assurance Committee. Literature review of the usefulness of nerve conduction studies and electromyography for the evaluation of patients with carpal tunnel syndrome. *Muscle & nerve*, 1993, *16*(12), 1392-1414.

Jenmalm, P; Dahlstedt, S; Johansson, RS. Visual and tactile information about object-curvature control fingertip forces and grasp kinematics in human dexterous manipulation. *J Neurophysiol*, 2000, 84, 2984–2997.

Jenmalm, P; Johansson, RS. Visual and somatosensory information about object shape control manipulative fingertip forces. *J Neurosci*, 1997, 17(11), 4486-99.

Johansson, RS. Sensory input and control of grip. *Sensory guidance of movement*. Wiley, Chichester (Novartis Foundation Symposium 218), 45-63, 1998.

Johansson, RS. Somatosensory signals and sensorimotor transformations in reactive control of grasp. In: Franzen O, Johansson R and Terenius L, eds. *Somesthesis and the Neurobiology of the Somatosensory Cortex.* Birkhauser Verlag Basel, 271-82, 1996.

Johansson, RS; Cole, KJ. (1994). Grasp stability during manipulative actions. *Can J Physiol Pharmacol.*, 72, 511–524.

Johansson, RS; Flanagan, JR. Coding and use of tactile signals from the fingertips in object manipulation tasks. *Nat Rev Neurosci*, 2009, 10, 345–359.

Johansson, RS; Westling, G. Roles of glabrous skin receptors and sensorimotor memory in automatic control of precision grip when lifting rougher or more slippery objects. *Exp Brain Res*, 1984, 56, 550-64.

Johansson, RS; Westling, G. Signals in tactile afferents from the fingers eliciting adaptive motor responses during precision grip. *Exp Brain Res*, 1987, 66, 141-54.

Johansson, RS; Westling, G. Coordinated isometric muscle commands adequately and erroneously programmed for the weight during lifting task with precision grip. *Exp Brain Res*, 1988a, 71, 59-71.

Johansson, RS; Westling, G. Programmed and triggered reactions to rapid load changes during precision. *Exp Brain Res*, 1988b, 71, 72-86.

Kanaan, N; Sawaya, RA. Carpal tunnel syndrome: modern diagnostic and management techniques. *Br J Gen Pract*, 2001, 51: 311–314.

Kimura, J. *Electrodiagnosis in Diseases of Nerve and Muscle: Principles and Practice*, ed 3. New York: Oxford University Press., 2001.

Kiser, D. Physiological and biomechanical factors for understanding repetitive motion injuries., *Sem Occup Med*, 1987, 2, 11–17

Li, ZM; Tang, J; Chakan, M; Kaz, R. Carpal tunnel expansion by palmarly directed forces to the transverse carpal ligament. *Journal of biomechanical engineering*, 2009, *131*(8), 081011.

Macefield, VG; Hager-Ross, C; Johansson, RS. Control of grip force during restraint of an object held between finger and thumb: responses of cutaneous afferents from the digits. *Exp Brain Res*, 1996, 108(1), 155-71.

Massy-Westropp; N, Grimmer; K, Bain; G. A systematic review of the clinical diagnostic tests for carpal tunnel syndrome. *The Journal of hand surgery*, 2000, 25(1), 120-127.

Moberg, E. Criticism and study of methods for examining sensibility in the hand. *Neurol*, 1962, 12, 8–19.

Mondelli, M; Padua, L; Reale, F. Carpal tunnel syndrome in elderly patients: results of surgical decompression. *J Peripher Nerv Syst*, 2004, 9(3), 168-76.

Monzee, J; Lamarre, Y; Smith, AM. The effects of digital anesthesia on force control using a precision grip. J *Neurophysiol*, 2003, 89(2), 672-83.

Newell, KM. Motor skill acquisition. *Annu Rev Psychol*, 1991, 42, 213–37.

Nora, DB; Becker, J; Ehlers, JA; Gomes, I: Clinical features of 1039 patients with neurophysiological diagnosis of carpal tunnel syndrome. *Clin Neurol Neurosurg*, 2004, 107, 64–69.

Nowak, DA; Glasauer, S; Hermsdorfer J. (2003) Grip force efficiency in long-term deprivation of somatosensory feedback. *Neuroreport*, 14, 1803–1807.

Oh, SJ. Clinical Electromyography: Nerve Conduction Studies, ed. 2. Baltimore, MD: Williams & Wilkins., 1993.

Oh SJ. Principles of Clinical Electromyography: Case Studies. Philadelphia, PA: Lippincott Williams & Wilkins., 1998.

Oh, SJ. Electrophysiologic tests in neuromuscular diseases. In: Pourmand R, ed. Neuromuscular Diseases: Expert Clinicians' Views. *Boston, MA: Butterworth Heinemann*. 1–49., 2001.

Oh SJ. *Clinical Electromyography: Nerve Conduction Studies*, ed 3. Philadelphia, PA: Lippincott, Williams & Wilkins., 2003.

Prilutsky BI. Coordination of two-and one-joint muscles: functional consequences and implications for motor control. *Motor Control*, 2000, 4, 1–44.

Rearick, MP; Casares, A; Santello, M. Task-dependent modulation of multi-digit force coordination patterns. *J Neurophys*, 2003, 89(3), 1317-26.

Rearick, MP; Santello, M. Force synergies for multifingered grasping. Effect of predictability in object center of mass and handedness. *Exp Br Res*, 2002, 44, 38-49.

Rearick, MP; Stelmach, GE; Leis, B; Santello, M. Coordination and control of forces during multifingered grasping in Parkinson's disease. *Exp Neurol*, 2002, 177, 428-42.

Reilmann, R; Gordon, AM; Henningsen, H. Initiation and development of fingertip forces during wholehand grasping. *Exp Br Res*, 2001, 140, 443-52.

Salimi, I; Frazier, W; Reilmann, R; Gordon AM. Selective use of visual information signaling objects' center of mass for anticipatory control of manipulative fingertip forces. *Exp Br Res*, 2003, 150, 9-18.

Salimi, I; Hollender, I; Frazier, W; Gordon, AM. Specificity of internal representations underlying grasping. *J Neurophysiol*, 2000, 84, 2390-7.

Santello, M; Soechting, JF. Force synergies for multifingered grasping. *Exp Br Res*, 2000, 133, 457-67.

Siegel, DB; Kuzma, G; Eakins, D. Anatomic investigation of the role of the lumbrical muscles in carpal tunnel syndrome. *J Hand Surg*, 1995; 20, 860-3.

Silverstein, BA; Fine, LJ; Armstrong, TJ. Occupational factors and carpal tunnel syndrome. *American journal of industrial medicine*, 1987, *11*(3), 343-358.

Smith, MA; Soechting, JF. Modulation of grasping forces during object transport. *J Neurophys*, 2005, 93, 137-145.

Thonnard, J-L; Saels, P; Van den Bergh, P; Lejeune, T. Effects of chronic median nerve compression at the wrist on sensation and manual skills. *Exp Br Res*, 1999, 128, 61–64.

Tinazzi; M, Zanette; G, Volpato; D, Testoni; R, Bonato; C, Manganotti; P., Miniussi, C, Fiaschi; A. (1998). Neurophysiological evidence of neuroplasticity at multiple levels of the somatosensory system in patients with carpal tunnel syndrome. *Brain*, 1998, *121*(9), 1785-1794.

Ugbolue, UC; Hsu, WH; Goitz, RJ; Li, ZM. Tendon and nerve displacement at the wrist during finger movements. *Clinical Biomechanics*, 2005, *20*(1), 50-56.

Verdugo; RJ; Salinas; RA; Castillo; JL, Cea; JG. Surgical versus non-surgical treatment for carpal tunnel syndrome. *Cochrane Database Syst Rev*, 2008, 4.

Vereijken, B; Van Emmerick, REA; Writing, HTA; Newell, KM: Free(z)ing degrees of freedom in skill acquisition. *J Mot Behav*, 1992, 24,133–142.

Welford, AT: Skill learning and performance. The obtaining and processing of information: some basic issues relating to analysing inputs and making decisions. *Res Q* 1972, 43, 295–311.

Westling, G; Johansson, RS. Factors influencing the force control during precision grip. *Exp Br Res*, 1984, 53, 277-284.

Wing, AM: More grip, less force. *Occup Health Saf*, 2006, 75, 68–72.

Witt, JC; Hentz, JG; Clarke, Stevens J. (2004). Carpal tunnel syndrome with normal nerve conduction studies. *Muscle Nerve*, 29. 515–522.

Wolpert, DM; Flanagan, JR. Motor prediction. *Curr Biol*, 2001, 11, 729–732.

Xiu, KH; Kim, JH; Li, ZM. Biomechanics of the transverse carpal arch under carpal bone loading. *Clinical Biomechanics*, 2010, 25(8), 776-780.

Yii, NW; Elliot, D. A study of the dynamic relationship of the lumbrical muscles and the carpal tunnel. *J Hand Surg*, 1994, 19, 439-43.

Zhang, W; Gordon, AM; Fu, Q; Santello, M. Manipulation after object rotation reveals independent sensorimotor memory representations of digit positions and forces. *Journal of neurophysiology*, 2010, 103(6), 2953-2964.

Zhang, W, Johnston, JA; Ross, MA; Smith, AA; Coakley, BJ; Gleason, EA; Dueck, AC; Santello, M. Effects of carpal tunnel syndrome on adaptation of multi-digit forces to object weight for whole-hand manipulation. *PLoS One*, 2011, 6(11), e27715.

Zhang, W, Johnston, JA; Ross, MA; Smith, AA; Coakley, BJ; Gleason, EA; Dueck, AC; Santello, M. Effects of Carpal Tunnel Syndrome on adaptation of multi-digit forces to object mass distribution for whole-hand manipulation. *J Neuroeng Rehabil*, 2012, 9, 83.

Zhang, W, Johnston, JA; Ross, MA; Sanniec, K; Gleason, EA; Dueck, AC; Santello, M. Effects of carpal tunnel syndrome on dexterous manipulation are grip type-dependent. *PLoS One*, 2013, 8(1), e53751.

In: Carpal Tunnel Syndrome
Editor: Morton Ledford

Chapter 4

Assessment of Carpal Tunnel Syndrome: Overview of Clinical Tests

Carla Vanti, PT, OMT, MSc[*]
and Paolo Pillastrini, PT, MSc[†]

Department of Biomedical and Neuromotor Sciences (DIBINEM),
Alma Mater Studiorum, University of Bologna, Bologna, Italy

Abstract

Study design. Narrative review of diagnostic studies.

Introduction. Carpal tunnel syndrome (CTS) is one of the most common pathologies of the peripheral nervous system. Several clinical tests have been proposed to diagnose CTS, despite the fact that their psychometric properties continue to be disputed. The aim of this contribution is to collect, through a narrative review of literature, scientific evidence on the accuracy (reliability and validity) of diagnostic tests in CTS, and summarize current knowledge.

Methods. Research was carried out in the main biomedical electronic databases (PubMed, PEDro, EMBASE, CINAHL, Cochrane

---

[*] Corresponding Author: Carla Vanti PT, OMT, MSc, Department of Biomedical and Neuromotor Sciences (DIBINEM), Alma Mater Studiorum, University of Bologna, Bologna 40138, Italy, carla.vanti@unibo.it, Phone/Fax: +39 051 785254 Mobile: +39 335 475464
[†] Email: paolo.pillastrini@unibo.it, Phone/Fax: +39 051 6362496 Mobile: +39 338 9841588

Library). The following key words were used: "Carpal tunnel syndrome", "Physical examination", "Nerve conduction testing", "Median neuropathy", "Tension test", "Diagnostic testing", with no limits of date and in English, Spanish, Portuguese, French and Italian.

Results. This review concerns the following assessment tools: the Hand Diagram, the Inspection, the Neurological Exam, Tinel's test, Phalen's and Phalen's reverse tests, the Pressure Provocation Tests, the Upper Limb Neurodynamic Tests, and clusters of tests. Other tests such as the Tethered Median Nerve Stress test, the Hand elevation test, the Flick sign, the Closed Fist Sign, and the Tourniquet test are less used in clinical practice. The rates of reliability and diagnostic accuracy of various tests commonly used in CTS appear conflicting.

Conclusion. To make the correct diagnosis, it is advisable to use a cluster of tests rather than a single test. The development of "clinical prediction rules" may be one of the most interesting perspectives for the diagnosis of CTS.

Introduction

Carpal tunnel syndrome (CTS) is one of the most common nerve compression disorders, mainly affecting women aged 55 and older [1]. According to the Consensus Criteria for the Classification of CTS published by Rempel et al. [2], the typical symptoms of CTS include pain associated with numbness, tingling or burning in at least one of the first, second or third digits.

Epidemiological studies have shown that the incidence and prevalence of CTS in the general population can range respectively from 0.12% to 1% and from 5% to 16%, in relation to the different diagnostic criteria [3,4,5,6,7,8]. The prevalence of occupational CTS is highly variable, ranging from 0.6 to 61%, depending on the various professional categories considered [9]. Clinical diagnosis of CTS is usually derived from a combination of clinical symptoms, signs and median nerve conduction studies (NCS). Although discrepancies between CTS clinical symptoms and NCS abnormalities are widely reported both in the general population [10,11] and in working populations [12,13], a report from the American Association of Electrodiagnostic Medicine [14] recommends nerve conduction studies to confirm a clinical diagnosis of CTS, with a high degree of sensitivity and specificity [15,16]. Therefore, NCS are still the reference standard for CTS diagnosis.

CTS symptoms usually begin with tingling, paresthesia and dysesthesia, followed by pain, especially at night. Symptoms occur in/are present in the first three digits of the hand, and occasionally in the fourth digit. In about a third of subjects, weakness and/or hypo/atrophy of the thenar eminence muscles appear, resulting in reduction or loss of grip strength between the thumb and forefinger. The inability to grasp small objects can be attributed to reduced sensitivity (hypoesthesia, anaesthesia) as well as the inability to oppose the thumb to the other fingers for muscular deficits. Patients may also report pain radiating to the forearm, elbow or even shoulder.

The most common subjective symptom is paresthesia or an unpleasant sensation of tingling or numbness at night, which can disrupt sleep and is often associated with pain. Paresthesia is typically attenuated by changing the position of the arm, vigorous movement, or hand massage. In some cases, subjects adopt some relieving strategies such as leaving their hand inclined downwards, out of the bed, or dipping the affected limb in cold water. Paresthesia may also occur during the day and is often triggered by sustained positions or activities such as driving, sewing, writing, washing dishes, ironing [6, 17, 18].

CTS can present as acute or chronic. The acute form is less common and is caused by a sudden and significant increase of pressure in the carpal tunnel. This condition is often associated with traumatic events such as a radius fracture, subluxation of the carpal tunnel, local infection or inflammation of the wrist. Acute forms may also occur as a result of immobilizing the wrist with rigid braces or splints (i.e. after Colles' fracture). The Cotton-Loder position, characterized by wrist flexion, is used to reduce and stabilize fractures of the distal radius, however it has been shown to increase pressure in the carpal tunnel [19]. The chronic CTS form, which is the most common and widespread, is characterized by an insidious onset and a persistence of symptoms for months or years.

Symptoms of CTS are related to increased mechanosensitivity, although there may be differences between acute and chronic presentations. Acute compression can provoke inflammation and neural irritation [20]. The increased intra-carpal canal pressure changes the microcirculation up to complete ischemia [21]. Acute ischemia may cause acute and intermittent paresthesias, that reflect ectopic impulse generation in large myelinated sensory fibers due to a transient disruption of membrane excitability [22].

In chronic CTS, the biological response of the nerve is similar and characterized by perineural edema, followed by short-term macrophage recruitment and fibrosis [21, 23]. Neural irritation and subsequent increased mechanosensitivity may also occur in chronic CTS, especially if acute nerve compression and ischemia are superimposed on chronic nerve compression.

Given the socio-economic impact of CTS on the population and the relevance of medicolegal issues related to occupational factors, formulating the correct diagnosis is crucial. Several clinical tests have been proposed to diagnose this syndrome, despite the fact that their psychometric properties continue to be disputed. The aim of this contribution is to collect, through a narrative review of literature, scientific evidence on the accuracy (reliability and validity) of diagnostic tests in CTS, and summarize current knowledge.

Materials and Methods

Research was carried out in the main biomedical electronic databases (PubMed, PEDro, EMBASE, CINAHL, Cochrane Library). The following key words were used: "Carpal tunnel syndrome", "Physical examination", "Nerve conduction testing", "Median neuropathy", "Tension test", "Diagnostic testing", with no limits of date and in English, Spanish, Portuguese, French and Italian.

The results were organized in different paragraphs, concerning the main assessment tools, excluding nerve conduction studies, which are outside of the subject of this review.

Results

Anamnesis and Hand Diagram

Given the relevance of symptoms in diagnosing CTS, history provides important information about the patient's medical condition and possible associated diseases. Table 1 shows the common symptoms and the provocative or relieving factors increasing the likelihood of CTS [24], whereas Table 2 shows the reliability of the most common questions in patients with CTS [25]. From a clinical point of view, some old studies [17, 18] established that the presence of nocturnal paresthesia in CTS has sensitivity between 51% and 96% and specificity between 27% and 68%. Other more recent studies [26, 27, 28, 29] have shown conflicting results (Table 3), thus this subjective symptom can be considered disputable for the diagnosis of CTS, having shown a positive likelihood ratio (+LR) =1.2 and a negative likelihood ratio (-LR) =0.7 [30].

A high percentage of patients is initially unable to locate and properly describe what part of their hand or fingers is affected by paresthesia and they often refer symptoms in the whole hand, both on the dorsal and palmar aspects. However, some tools (provocative tests and self-assessment tests) help patients to better localize their symptoms. The diagram of the hand, or Katz Hand Diagram is a self-completed diagram, which represents the dorsal and palmar aspects of the hands. Patients can use this diagram to mark the location and the quality (tingling, numbness, pain, etc.) of their symptoms. According to the Consensus Criteria indicated by Katz et al. [29] and by Rempel et al. [2], subjects are classified, for the right hand and for the left hand, as follows:

a   classic CTS= symptoms in at least two of digits 1-3; may have symptoms in digits 4-5, wrist pain, proximal radiation of pain; palm or dorsum cannot be affected;
b   probable CTS = same, except palmar symptoms allowed, unless only on ulnar border;
c   possible CTS = symptoms only in one of digits 1-3.
d   unlikely CTS = no symptoms in digits 1-3.

Priganc & Henry [31] showed that the hand diagram is highly reliable (0.95) if compared to the grade of severity of CTS and a metanalysis from D'Arcy and McGee [30] concluded that a classic or probable diagram is indicative of CTS with sensitivity = 64%, specificity = 73%, +LR=2.4, and -LR=0.5. The results of individual studies on the hand diagram are shown in Table 4.

Table 1. Symptoms, provocative and relieving factors increasing the likelihood of CTS. Modified from: Colombini D et al. Le affezioni muscoloscheletriche degli arti superiori e inferiori come patologie professionali; quali e a quali condizioni. Documento di consenso di un gruppo di lavoro nazionale. Med Lav. 2003;94(3):312–329 [24]

Common symptoms
Dull aching discomfort in the hand, forearm, or upper arm
Hand paresthesia
Weakness or clumsiness in the hand
Dry skin, swelling or colour changes of the hand
Occurrence of these symptoms in the median distribution

Table 1. (Continued)

Provocative factors
Sleep
Sustained arm or hand positions
Repetitive actions of the hand and wrist
Relieving factors
Change in hand posture
Shaking of the hand

Table 2. Reliability of the questions in CTS. Modified from: Wainner RS et al. Development of a clinical prediction rule for the diagnosis of carpal tunnel syndrome. Arch Phys Med Rehabil. 2005;86:609-18 [25]

Question	Reliability K Coefficient (IC 95%)
Which of the following symptoms are most bothersome for you?	K= 0.74 (0.55, 0.93)
Where are your symptoms most bothersome?	K=0.82 (0.68, 0.96)
Which of the following best describes the behavior of your symptoms?	K=0.57 (0.35,0.79)
Does your affected hand feel "fat" or "swollen"?	K=0.85 (0.68, 1.0)
Do you have trouble with fumbling or dropping objects from your affected hand?	K=0.95 (0.85, 1.0)
Does your entire affected limb and/or hand feel numb?	K=0.53 (0.26, 0.81)
Do your symptoms wake you during the night?	K=0.83 (0.60, 1.0)
Do your symptoms improve with moving, "shaking," or positioning your wrist or hands?	K=0.90 (0.75, 1.0)
Are your symptoms made worse when performing tasks that require a lot of grasping or hand and/or finger use?	K=0.72 (0.49, 0.95)

Table 3. Diagnostic accuracy of nocturnal paresthesias. Modified from: Cook Ch.E, Hegedus EJ. Orthopedic Physical Examination Tests: An Evidence-Based Approach (2nd Edition). Pearson Education Inc, 2013 [40]

Author	Sensitivity	Specificity	+lr	-LR
Buch-Jaeger et al. [26]	51	68	1.6	0.7
Gupta et al. [27]	84	33	1.2	0.5
Katz et al. [29]	77	27	1.1	0.8
Szabo et al. [28]	96	100	Not applicable	0.04

The studies are in alphabetical order by author.

Table 4. Diagnostic accuracy of the Katz Hand Diagram. Modified from: Cook Ch.E, Hegedus EJ. Orthopedic Physical Examination Tests: An Evidence-Based Approach (2nd Edition). Pearson Education Inc., 2013 [40]

Author	Sensitivity	Specificity	+LR	-LR
Atroshi et al. [1]	80	90	8.0	0.2
Gunnarsonn et al. [82]	66	69	2.1	0.5
Katz & Stirrat [83]	80	90	3.6	0.1
Katz et al. [84]	61	71	2.1	0.5
O' Gradaigh & Merry[85]	72	53	1.5	0.5
Szabo et al. [28]	76	98	38.0	0.2

The studies are in alphabetical order by author.

Physical Exam

The physical examination is the second part of the patient's assessment and includes an inspection, a neurological exam, and provocative tests.

Inspection

Inspecting the skin is a significant part of the physical exam. In CTS, the skin may appear pale and drier than normal, sometimes with excessive sweating and/or dark in color. Generally the skin appears smooth and thin, but in the case of long-term nerve damage, it is rough, inelastic and dry; nails can be curved, grooved and tapered. The skin inspection may show also a simultaneous presence of "Raynaud's phenomenon", which could raise the suspicion of scleroderma in the initial phase. It is also important to investigate the tropism of the hand muscles: in more advanced cases of CTS, hypotrophy or atrophy of the thenar eminence may be observed (+LR=1.6, -LR=1.0) [30]. In severe cases, characterized by paralysis of the median nerve, you can see a posture of a "hand raised in blessing" or "preacher hand." [32].

Some authors have proposed the so-called *"Square wrist sign"*, which is obtained by measuring the anterior-posterior and medium-lateral diameters of the wrist with an adjustable compass. Clinical studies report sensitivity of this test from 47% to 69% and specificity from 73% to 83% [33,34]. Generally, the square wrist sign demonstrates moderate diagnostic accuracy (+LR=2.7, -

LR=0.5) [30]. If the ratio between the anterior-posterior and medium-lateral diameters of the wrist is greater than 0.70 and abductor pollicis brevis is weak, these two signs are moderately sensitive [33]. Moreover, Wainner included this sign in a cluster of tests to predict CTS [25].

Neurological Exam

The **clinical sensitivity exam** in the median nerve territory should be accurate, logical and systematic, going from proximal to distal and including all the possible sensory modalities: tactile, thermal, pain, vibratory, proprioceptive, discriminative [35]. This examination should not be limited to merely detecting the presence or absence of sensitivity, but should also recognize subtle differences in sensitivity and the presence of paresthesia and dysesthesia. The two hands should be compared and the differences between the first three digits and the fifth digit (which is innervated by the ulnar nerve) should be assessed on the affected hand.

- *Tactile sensitivity exam* – Changes in light touch are generally assessed using a needle, a cotton swab or an algesimeter. The finding of hypalgesia in the median nerve territory is relevant for diagnosis (+LR=3.1), but if the result is negative, we cannot exclude CTS (-LR=0.7) [30].

Other possible sensitivity exams are the Semmes-Weinstein test (threshold test using a monofilament), the vibratory sensitivity test (using a tuning fork) and the discrimination of two points (innervation density test).

- *Semmes-Weinstein test* – It is executed placing a thin needle perpendicular to the palmar surface of the patient's hand and gradually applying pressure until the needle tends to curve. This test is positive if the patient, with his/her eyes closed, cannot recognize pressure corresponding to 2.83 milligrams. This test has shown scarce reliability (0.22) [36] and highly variable diagnostic accuracy among different authors.
- *Vibratory sensitivity test* - A 256 oscillation-per-second tuning fork is struck against a stationary object and then placed on the patient's fingertip. Each finger is tested and compared with the contralateral one. The test is positive if the perception of the stimulus is perceived

as different compared to the contralateral one. The reliability of this test between two examiners was measured as 0.71 [36], whereas its diagnostic accuracy is highly different among various studies.

- *Discrimination of two points* - The patient is required to identify the minimum distance from two separate pressure points, the 6 mm cut-off is commonly used. The discrimination of two points has shown low sensitivity and high specificity. Both Massy-Westropp et al. [37], and D'Arcy and McGee [30] in their systematic reviews concluded that its diagnostic validity is scarce (+LR=1.3, and –LR=1.0).

The clinical muscular exam is aimed at testing the muscle strength of individual muscles or groups of muscles innervated by the median nerve to estimate the stage of CTS with good approximation. For a rapid test, the function of the abductor pollicis brevis, located superficially on the radial aspect of the thenar mass, is assessed. Weakness of the abductor pollicis brevis muscle demonstrates moderate diagnostic accuracy for CTS (+LR=1.8, -LR=0.5) and fair reliability (0.25) [38]. However, it is appropriate to test all the hand muscles innervated by the median nerve: the abductor pollicis brevis, the opponens pollicis, the flexor pollicis longus, the flexor pollicis brevis (superficial portion), the flexor digitorum profundus (lateral portion), the flexor digitorum superficialis [6,28].

Provocative Tests

Several provocative tests have been described in CTS, with different levels of reliability and diagnostic accuracy [39,40]. First of all, we must point out that none of them alone is a diagnostic test because provocative tests aim only to reproduce CTS symptoms in the median nerve territory. As a consequence, the results of provocative tests should be considered complementary to the history, the neurological exam and the nerve conduction testing. More than one provocative test is commonly used in clinical practice, also involving other joints of the upper limb. The most frequently used provocative tests are: Tinel's test, Phalen's test, the Pressure Provocation tests, and the Tension tests of the median nerve (Upper Limb Neurodynamic Tests). Other tests, such as the Tethered Median Nerve Stress test, the Hand Elevation test, the Flick sign, the Closed fist sign and the Tourniquet test are used less in clinical practice.

Tinel's Test

Tinel first described this test in 1915, and it is one of the most investigated clinical tools for the diagnosis of CTS. It is still widely used in clinical practice, although several factors can influence its positivity. The patient's forearm is in supination and his/her wrist is in the dorsiflexion position. The examiner hits (with an examination hammer or with his/her fingers) the palmar surface of the wrist 4-6 times, distal to the wrist folds and laterally to the palmaris longus tendon. This is where the median nerve passes through the carpal tunnel (see Figure 1). This test is positive if it evokes paresthesia in the territory of the median nerve.

The first critical element of this test is the amount of pressure used: most discrepancies between different examiners can be thus attributed. On the other hand, it is difficult to quantify exactly how much pressure should be used, as the use of excessive force can produce paresthesia even on a normal nerve.

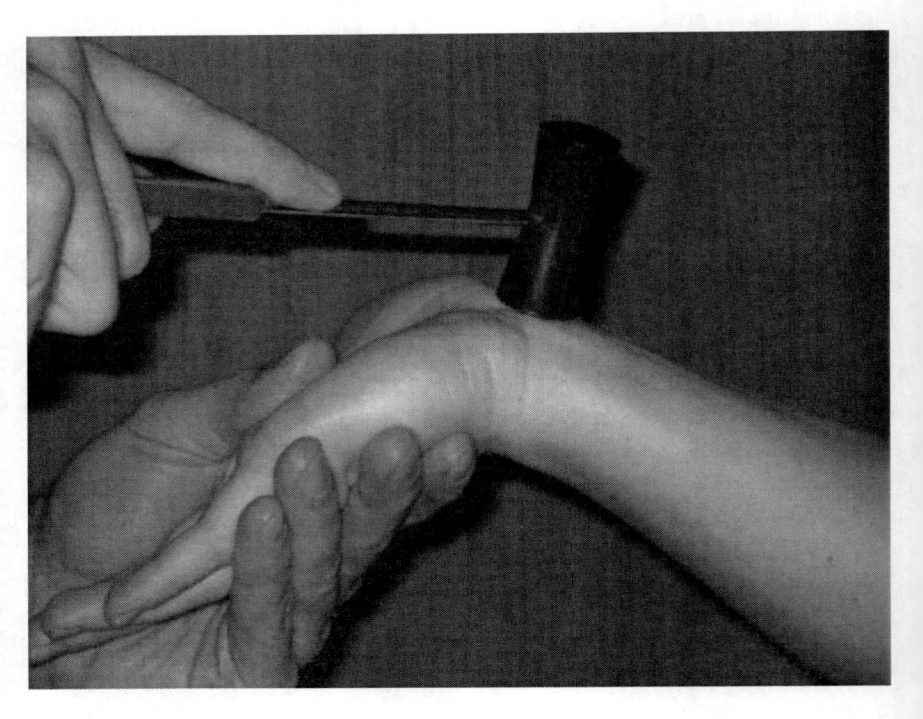

Figure 1. Tinel's Test.

Clinical studies have shown very different rates of diagnostic accuracy and several variations can be observed regarding the location and the number of percussions executed. The sensitivity of this test varies from 23% to 97%, specificity from 31% to 100%, and coefficients of reliability from 0.47 [25] to 0.81 [36]. (see Table 5)

It has been observed in several cases that Tinel's test can be positive even in the absence of any compressive pathologies. Kuschner et al. [41] and Mondelli et al. [42] conclude that Tinel's test alone is not sufficient to make a diagnosis of CTS, since it does not search for a combination of different signs, which would be more useful than a single sign. Despite the conflicting opinions of different authors, a review from Valdes & LaStayo [43], based on the quality of the studies and on the calculation of the +LS (=2.95) and –LR (=0.57), suggests this test as one of the most highly recommended provocative tests for CTS.

Table 5. Diagnostic accuracy of Tinel's Test. Modified from: Cook Ch.E, Hegedus EJ. Orthopedic Physical Examination Tests: An Evidence-Based Approach (2nd Edition). Pearson Education Inc, 2013 [40]

Author	Sensitivity	Specificity	+LR	-LR
Ahn [7]	68	90	6.8	0.4
Amirfeyz et al. [72]	48	94	8.0	0.6
Amirfeyz et al. [73]	53	93	7.45	0.51
Borg et al. [86]	64	62	1.7	0.6
Brüske et al. [87]	67	68	2.09	0.49
Buch-Jaeger et al. [26]	42	64	1.1	0.9
Cheng et al. [88]	32	99	32	0.69
De Krom et al. [45]	35	53	0.7	1.2
Durkan [89]	56	80	2.8	0.6
Gellmann et al. [77]	44	94	7.3	0.6
Gelmers [90]	43	74	1.7	0.8
Gerr et al. [91]	25	67	0.7	1.1
Golding et al. [76]	26	80	1.3	0.9
Gonzales del Pino et al. [92]	33	97	11	0.7
Gunnarsonn et al. [82]	62	57	1.4	0.7
Hansen et al. [93]	27	91	3.0	0.8
Heller et al. [94]	60	77	2.7	0.5
Katz et al. [84]	59	67	1.8	0.6
Kuhlman et al. [33]	23	87	1.8	0.9
LaJoie et al. [95]	97	91	11	0.03
MacDermid et al. [36]	59-41	92-94	7.4-6.8	0.5-0.6

Table 5. (Continued)

Author	Sensitivity	Specificity	+LR	-LR
El Miedany et al. [96]	30	65	0.86	1.08
Mondelli et al. [5]	41	90	4.1	0.7
O'Gradaigh et al. [85]	55	72	2.0	0.6
Seror [97]	63	45	1.1	0.8
Stewart et al. [98]	40	71	1.4	0.8
Szabo et al. [28]	64	99	64	0.4
Tetro et al. [47]	74	91	8.2	0.3
Wainner et al. [99]	41	58	0.98	1.01
Walters & Rice [100]	64-57	40-31	1.1-0.8	0.9-1.4
Williams et al. [46]	67	100	NA	0.3
Yii et al. [75]	42	100	NA	0.6

The studies are in alphabetical order by author.

Phalen's Test

This test was first described in 1957 by Phalen and Kendrick [44]. The patient is asked to hold the dorsal aspects of his/her hands together for about a minute, keeping his/her elbows in full flexion and his/her forearms in a horizontal position (see Figure 2). Wrist flexion causes the compression of the median nerve in the carpal tunnel between the transverse carpal ligament and the finger flexor tendons. The test is considered positive if symptoms in the territory of the median nerve (in particular on the first three digits of the hand) are evoked. Patients with advanced stage CTS often report the onset of paresthesia in less than 20 seconds.

The sensitivity of this test, as reported by various authors, ranges from 10% to 92%, specificity from 33% to 100% (see Table 6), inter-examiner reliability was rated =0.79 [25] and relationship with the severity of CTS =0.58 [31]. Some authors modified this test, varying the position of the wrist or the elbow, including external pressure on the dorsal aspects of the hands, or adding passive wrist flexion applied by the examiner. Despite the conflicting opinions of different authors, the review from Valdes & LaStayo [43] also suggests this test as one of the most highly recommended provocative tests for CTS (+LR=2.68, -LR=0.54), especially for moderate and severe CTS.

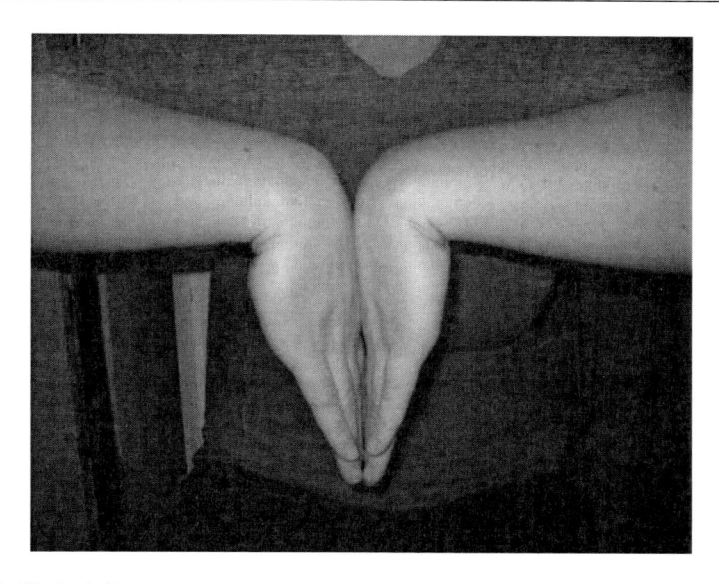

Figure 2. Phalen's Test.

Table 6. Diagnostic accuracy of Phalen's Test. Modified from: Cook Ch.E, Hegedus EJ. Orthopedic Physical Examination Tests: An Evidence-Based Approach (2nd Edition). Pearson Education Inc., 2013 [40]

Author	Sensitivity	Specificity	+lr	-lr
Ahn [71]	68	91	7.4	0.4
Amirfeyz et al. [72]	83	98	41.5	0.17
Amirfeyz et al. [73]	87	84	5.55	0.15
Boland et al. [101]	64	75	2.54	0.49
Borg et al. [86]	83	67	2.5	0.3
Brüske et al. [87]	85	89	7.73	0.17
Buch-Jaeger et al. [26]	58	54	1.3	0.8
Burke et al. [102]	51	54	1.1	0.9
De Krom et al. [4]	49	48	0.9	1.1
De Smet et al. [103]	91	33	1.4	0.3
Durkan [104]	70	84	4.4	0.4
Fertl et al. [105]	79	92	9.9	0.2
Gellmann et al. [77]	71	80	3.6	0.4
Gerr et al. [91]	75	33	1.1	0.7

Table 6. (Continued)

Author	Sensitivity	Specificity	+LR	-LR
Golding et al. [76]	10	86	0.7	1.0
Gonzalez del Pino et al. [92]	87	90	8.7	0.1
Gunnarsonn et al. [82]	86	48	1.7	0.3
Hansen et al. [93]	34	74	1.3	0.9
Heller et al. [94]	67	59	1.6	0.6
Katz et al. [83]	75	47	1.4	0.5
Kuhlman et al. [33]	51	76	2.1	0.6
LaJoie et al. [95]	92	88	7.7	0.1
El Miedany et al. [96]	47	17	0.57	3.12
Mondelli et al. [42]	59	93	8.4	0.4
O'Gradaigh et al. [85]	72	53	1.5	0.5
Seror [97]	62	90	6.2	0.42
Szabo et al. [28]	75	95	15	0.3
Tetro et al. [47]	61	83	3.6	0.5
Wainner et al. [99]	77	40	1.29	0.58
Williams et al. [46]	88	100	NA	0.12
Yii et al. [75]	87	93	12	0.1

Reverse Phalen's Test

The execution of this test is similar to the conventional Phalen's Test but instead of wrist flexion, maximum wrist extension is required for about one minute, thereby stretching the median nerve. In addition, the examiner can apply slight pressure with his/her thumb on the carpal tunnel, compressing it further.

Only few studies have investigated this test, which is not strongly recommended [43]. Its sensitivity can vary from 41% [45] to 75% and specificity from 0.35 to 0.96; its reliability was calculated by Mac Dermid et al. (K=0.72).

Pressure Provocation Tests (Median Nerve Compression Test, Median Nerve Compression Test and Wrist Flexion, Carpal Compression Test, Modified Carpal Compression Test)

Median Nerve Compression Test - With the patient's wrist extended, the examiner grasps the patient's wrist with both hands and exerts pressure directly on the median nerve (under the flexor retinaculum, between the flexor carpi radialis and palmaris longus muscles) with both his/her thumbs, for 15 seconds to two minutes. This test is positive if the patient's known symptoms (pain, paresthesia, numbness) are reproduced and if these symptoms are relieved when pressure is released. Some studies (see Table 7) have shown sensitivity from 42% to 100%, specificity from 68% to 100%, and reliability =0.92 [46].

Table 7. Diagnostic accuracy of the Median Nerve Compression Test. Modified from: Cook Ch.E, Hegedus EJ. Orthopedic Physical Examination Tests: An Evidence-Based Approach (2nd Edition). Pearson Education Inc, 2013 [40]

Author	Sensitivity	Specificity	+LR	-LR
Kaul et al. [70]	55	68	1.7	0.7
Mondelli et al. [42]	42	99	42	0.6
Williams et al. [46]	100	97	33	NA
Yii et al. [75]	81	100	NA	0.2

The studies are in alphabetical order by author.

Median Nerve Compression Test and Wrist flexion - With the patient's elbow flexed, forearm supinated and wrist flexed at 60°, the examiner grasps the patient's wrist with both hands and exerts sustained pressure directly on the median nerve with both his/her thumbs. This test is positive if the patient's known symptoms are reproduced within 30 seconds. Tetro et al. [47] proposed this test, that showed sensitivity =86%, specificity =95%, +LR=17, and −LR=0.1. This test is highly suggested in the systematic review by Massy-Westropp et al. [37], because it demonstrates high sensitivity and specificity.

Carpal Compression Test - With the patient's wrist extended, the examiner grasps the patient's wrist with both hands and exerts direct pressure on the carpal tunnel with both his/her thumbs for 30-60 seconds. Applying mechanical pressure on the carpal tunnel provokes an increase in pressure on the median nerve (see Figure 3). This test is positive if the patient's known symptoms are reproduced (paresthesia, numbness).

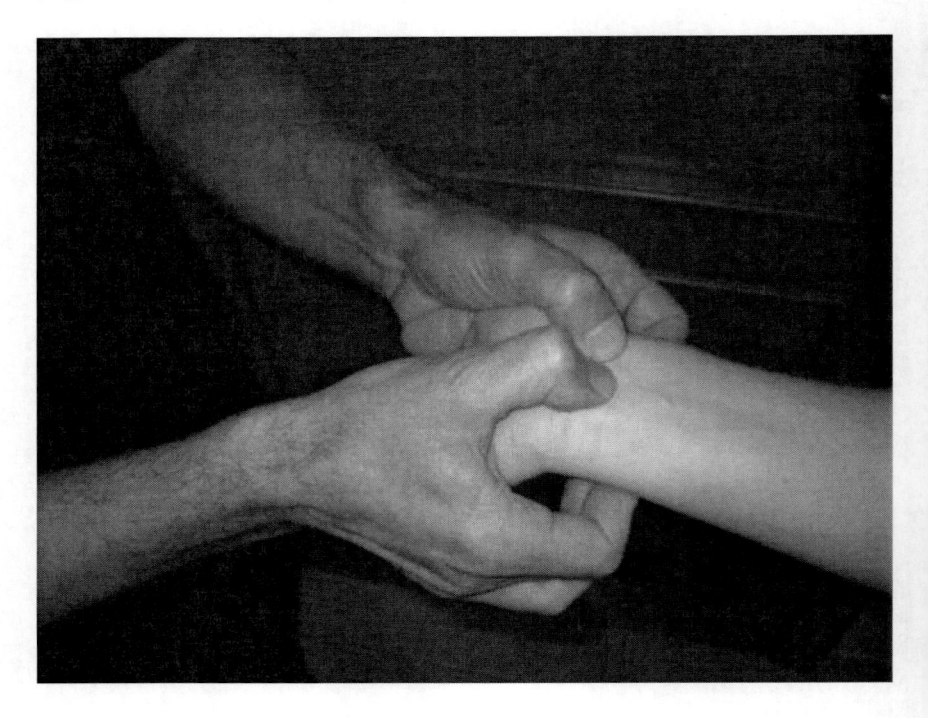

Figure 3. Carpal tunnel compression test.

Different studies reported sensitivity from 5% to 89%, specificity from 25% to 99% (see Table 8) and K coefficient =0.77 [25]. Some authors applied this test with a shorter pressure time (from 5 to 20 seconds) or employing a pressure-specified sensory device to measure the exerted pressure precisely.

Modified Carpal Compression test - The modified carpal compression test follows the same principles, with a minor modification regarding the compression site. This modified compression test is suggested by Valdes & LaStayo [43], as one of the most highly recommended provocative tests for CTS (+LR=2.28, -LR=0.91).

Table 8. Diagnostic accuracy of the Carpal Tunnel Compression Test. Modified from: Cook Ch.E, Hegedus EJ. Orthopedic Physical Examination Tests: An Evidence-Based Approach (2nd Edition). Pearson Education Inc, 2013 [40]

Author	Sensitivity	Specificity	+LR	-LR
Amirfeyz et al. [73]	84	79	3.94	0.20
Buch-Jaeger et al. [26]	49	54	1.1	0.9
De Krom et al. [45]	5	94	0.8	1.0
Burke et al. [102]	52	38	0.8	1.3
De Smet et al. [103]	63	33	0.9	1.1
Durkan [89]	89	96	22	0.1
Durkan [104]	87	90	8.7	0.1
Fertl et al. [105]	83	92	10	0.2
Gonzalez del Pino et al. [92]	87	95	17	0.1
Kaul et al. [70]	53	62	1.4	0.8
Kuhlman et al. [33]	28	74	1.1	1.0
El Miedany et al. [96]	46	25	0.61	2.16
Szabo et al. [28]	89	91	9.9	0.1
Tekeoglu et al. [106]	82	98	41	0.18
Tetro et al. [47]	82	99	11	0.3
Wainner et al. [99]	36	57	0.8	1.1
Wainner et al. [64]	64	30	0.9	1.2

The studies are in alphabetical order by author.

Upper Limb Neurodynamic Tests

The provocative tests described so far aim to reproduce CTS symptoms through direct action on the carpal tunnel (like in the Pressure Provocation tests or in Tinel's test) or through indirect action via wrist extreme positions (like in Phalen's and reverse Phalen's tests). Another possibility to reproduce the patient's symptoms is provoking the median nerve within the carpal tunnel not only acting on the wrist joints, but also by moving other joints the median nerve crosses in its course. For these reasons, a provocative test that includes all the joints crossed by the median nerve might be more accurate than traditional tests used in CTS, which focus only on a single joint.

Neural Tissue Provocation or Neurodynamic Tests 'challenge the physical capabilities of the Nervous System by using multijoint movements of the limbs and/or trunk to alter the length and dimensions of the nerve bed surrounding corresponding neural structures' [48]. Upper Limb Neurodynamic Tests (ULNTs), as described by Butler, also called Upper Limb Tension Tests (ULTTs), move the neural tissues and stimulate them mechanically, providing insight into nerve structure mobility and tissue sensitivity to mechanical stresses [49]. Among these tests, ULNT1 in particular accentuates stress on the median nerve [50].

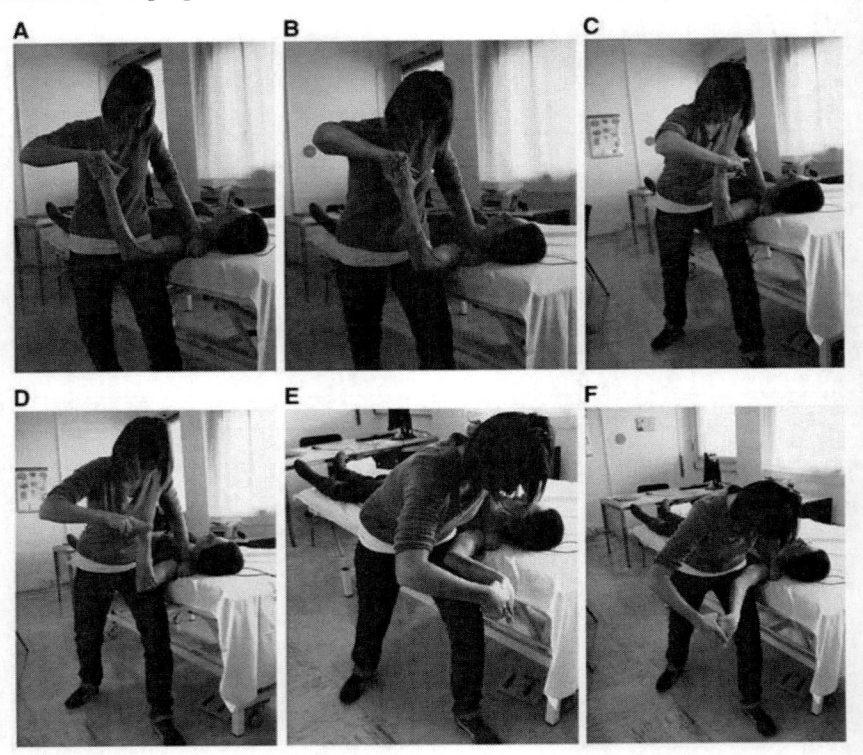

Figure 4. Stages of the ULNT1: (A) starting position; (B) shoulder abduction; (C) wrist extension; (D) forearm supination; (E) lateral shoulder rotation; and (F) elbow extension.

The involvement of other joints to elicit symptoms of neural origin is supported by anatomical studies, which show that tension can be transmitted at a distance in the peripheral nerves [51]. In the case of the median nerve, the shoulder and elbow joints are involved and the cervical spine is moved, because ipsilateral or contralateral cervical side bending alters median nerve longitudinal excursion [52]. Upper Limb Neurodynamic Test 1 (ULNT1) is executed in six steps. An example of this test on the left median nerve is shown in Figure 4.

1   The patient is supine, shifted on the side of the table ipsilateral to the arm to be tested. The examiner stands in front of the patient, with his/her right hand holding the patient's left hand, checking the patient's thumb and fingers. The patient's arm is in contact with the examiner's left thigh.

2   The examiner supports the patient's left fist on the table vertically, maintains the neutral position of the shoulder and prevents the shoulder girdle from elevating. The patient's arm is then abducted on the coronal plane at about 110°. Better arm support can be obtained by holding the patient's arm against the examiner's thigh during abduction.

3   Maintaining the obtained position, the patient's wrist and fingers are extended.

4   Maintaining the obtained position, the patient's forearm is supinated.

5   Maintaining the obtained position, the patient's shoulder is rotated externally.

6   Maintaining the obtained position, the patient's elbow is extended [53].

In this final position, cervical lateral flexions are added away from the tested side (in this example, on the right) and toward the tested side (in this example, on the left), to respectively increase and reduce tension on the median nerve [54]. This final part of the ULNT1 test is called "structural differentiation".

During this test, all patient symptoms are recorded. An important technical aspect to consider during neurodynamic testing is that each obtained position must be strictly maintained before adding another component of the test, otherwise the tension on the entire nerve may be dispersed. Any changes in symptoms, following a movement of a joint (in this case, the cervical spine) far from the site of the compression (in this case, the carpal tunnel) is not influenced by the tissues surrounding the carpal tunnel. This is an important aspect in differentiating symptoms of neural origin from local pathologies of the wrist such as arthritis, tendinitis, tenosynovitis and pain arising from a previous Colles' fracture.

There is no universally accepted procedure for this test, with regard to the sequence of movements (i.e. from proximal to distal, or vice-versa). Moreover, the positivity criteria of neurodynamic tests are not universally shared by all authors [55].

Nee and Butler [48] consider the test to be positive if: neural-mediated symptoms are reproduced, 'a movement of a body segment remote from the location of symptoms provoked in the neurodynamic test position alters the response', modifying the symptoms or the elbow extension (structural differentiation), 'if there are differences in the test response between the involved and uninvolved sides or variations from what is known to be a normal response in asymptomatic subjects'. Coppieters et al. [56] states that 'the neurodynamic test for the median nerve is considered positive in the diagnosis of CTS if neurogenic symptoms can be reproduced and if the intensity of the symptoms can be influenced by moving joints proximal to the wrist, while keeping the wrist position constant'.

Shacklock [49] states that the strongest indicator of an abnormal test is the reproduction of symptoms. However, he makes a distinction between an 'overt' abnormal response (characterized by the 'reproduction of symptoms and positive structural differentiation'), and a 'covert' abnormal response (i.e. 'a significant asymmetry of symptoms, symptoms in an abnormal location, loss of range of motion or a difference in palpable resistance to movement'). Nee et al. [57] states that 'a positive ULNT should at least partially reproduce the patient's symptoms and that structural differentiation should change these symptoms' [57].

Wainner et al. [25] considers the test as positive in the presence of at least one of the following: (1) reproduction of patient's symptoms; (2) side-to-side differences (>10°) in elbow extension on completion of all motion sequences; (3) symptomatic limb side: contralateral neck side bending increases symptoms or ipsilateral side bending decreases symptoms.

The intra- and inter-tester reliability of ULNT1 has been widely studied and ranges from moderate to good [25,58,59,60,61,62,63,64,65,66]. As far as diagnostic accuracy is concerned, Coveney et al. [67] found high sensitivity (82%), specificity (75%), +LR=3.29, and –LR=0.24 of ULNT1, whilst Wainner [25] found sensitivity =75%, specificity =13%, +LR=0.86, -LR=1.9, and reliability =0.76. Using Wainner's criteria for a positive test, Vanti et al. [50] found similar results (sensitivity =91%, specificity =15%, +LR=1.07, and –LR= 0.55). Mahmud et al. [68] showed a significant relationship (p=0,007) between the restriction of the range of motion (ROM) at the elbow during ULNT1 and electrophysiological alteration in 38 patients with CTS symptoms.

We can observe that the reproduction of symptoms in ULNT1 should be limited only to the portion of the median nerve implicated in CTS, in order to reduce false positives due to mechanical stimulation of other upper limb nerves (e.g. radial or ulnar nerve). Considering the reproduction of symptoms only in the thumb or lateral two fingers of the affected arm during ULNT1 as diagnostic criterion, diagnostic accuracy changed significantly. In two different studies, Vanti et al. confirmed weak diagnostic accuracy for CTS and specificity higher than sensitivity. In these studies, sensitivity ranged from 40% to 54%, specificity from 70% to 79%, +LR from 1.80 to 1.96, and –LR from 0.65 to 0.75 [50,55]. Including positive structural differentiation as mandatory criterion, specificity improved, but sensitivity decreased, thus the use of these additional criteria does not contribute to improving ULNT1 test performance [55].

Wainner also investigated the diagnostic accuracy of another neurodynamic test, called "Upper Limb Tension Test – part 2". With the patient supine and the shoulder abducted to 30°, the examiner sequentially introduced:

1   scapular depression,
2   medial shoulder rotation,
3   full elbow extension,
4   wrist and finger flexion,
5   contralateral then ipsilateral cervical side bending.

At each step of the test, the patient was questioned on symptom reproduction throughout the maneuver. The outcomes of this test were slightly inferior compared to ULNT1: inter-examiner reliability =0.83, sensitivity =64%, specificity =30%, +LR=1.2, and –LR=0.91.

In conclusion, the diagnostic accuracy of neurodynamic tests for CTS may be considered insufficient. From a clinical point of view, since neurodynamic tests challenge the physical capability of the nervous system according to the concept of "continuum", the presence of a positive neurodynamic test suggests increased mechanosensitivity of the neural tissue, but might not definitively indicate the specific site of nerve dysfunction [48,54]

Other Tests

Tethered Median Nerve Stress Test

With the patient's forearm supinated, the examiner hyperextends the index finger of the patient and consequently hyperextends his/her wrist, putting the median nerve entrapped at the wrist under tension. This test is positive if hand paresthesia or dysesthesia appear, with radiation to the volar surface of the forearm. This test was first proposed by LaBan [69] and then also investigated by Kaul et al. [70] and Mac Dermid et al. [36], showing sensitivity from 50% to 90%, specificity from 51% to 95%, and reliability of 0.49 [36].

Hand Elevation Test

This test is performed by asking the patient to raise both hands above his/her head and keep them raised until the onset of symptoms (paresthesia, numbness) in the territory of the median nerve. The test is positive if these symptoms appear within two minutes. Despite the fact that this test showed high diagnostic performance in a few studies [71,72,73], it is not commonly recommended [43]. Furthermore, we can note that same results could also appear in other clinical conditions, such as thoracic outlet syndrome.

Flick Sign

The "Flick sign" is elicited by asking the patient to reproduce a movement which usually relieves symptoms when they are severe or unbearable. The patient is asked to make a movement of the hand and wrist called the "flick", as if trying to shake a thermometer to reset it. This test is positive if symptoms, especially paresthesia, are reduced with this maneuver. Some differences among authors in this test concern the exact movement requested: either rapid alternating up and down movements of the wrist or even small movements of the elbow.

Table 9. Diagnostic accuracy of the Flick sign. Modified from: Cook Ch.E, Hegedus EJ. Orthopedic Physical Examination Tests: An Evidence-Based Approach (2nd Edition). Pearson Education Inc., 2013 [40]

Author	Sensitivity	Specificity	+LR	-LR
Pryse-Phillips [107]	93	96	23	0.1
Hansen et al. [93]	37	74	1.4	0.9
De Krom et al. [45]	50	61	1.3	0.8
Gunnarsson et al. [82]	90	30	1.3	0.3

The studies are in alphabetical order by author.

Table 9 summarizes the studies on the accuracy of this test. Despite the very different results of this test when applied alone, the Flick sign is cited as one of the five tests that compose the cluster proposed by Wainner et al. [25] and it is also recommended by Valdes & La Stayo [43].

Closed Fist Sign

The patient is asked to actively close the fingers into a fist for about 60 seconds. If CTS is present, lumbrical muscles are impaired in their possibility of sliding, and they can thus increase the pressure within the carpal tunnel. This test is positive if paresthesias in the territory of the median nerve are provoked. To the knowledge of the authors, no relevant evidence of accuracy has emerged from literature regarding this test [74,75].

Tourniquet Test

This test consists in placing a blood pressure cuff on the patient's arm, inflating up to just above the systolic pressure level and to keeping it inflated for about one minute. The test is positive if paresthesia or numbness in the territory of the median nerve are elicited. The rationale for this test is that a compressed median nerve is considered to be more susceptible to ischemia compared to a normal nerve. However, since even healthy subjects can complain about the onset of the same symptoms during this test, it is difficult to assess whether real CTS is present. Some studies [26,45,73,76,77] reported test sensitivity from 21% to 93% and specificity from 36% to 87%. Generally, low diagnostic accuracy supports the use of this test.

Cluster of Tests

As previously stated, no single test has been accepted as sufficient in itself to identify CTS in both clinical and research settings [36,45,78,79]. The scarce accuracy of these tests suggests that they may not be used as stand-alones and must be interpreted in combination with other clinical findings and diagnostic exams. For example, Szabo et al. [28] found that if a positive hand diagram was combined with night pain, abnormal sensitivity testing and positive carpal compression test, the probability of CTS was 86%.

Wainner et al. [25] developed a predictive pattern (clinical prediction rule - CPR) to clinically diagnose CTS. The clinical prediction rule identified in the Wainner study consisted of one question (shaking hands for symptom relief), wrist-ratio index greater than 0.67, Symptom Severity Scale score greater than

1.9, reduced median sensory in the territory of the first digit, and age greater than 45 years. The +LR for this CPR was 18.3 when all five tests were positive, indicating a great decisive change of probability that the patient had the pathology (see Table 10).

Table 10. Diagnostic accuracy of Wainner's Clinical Prediction Rule. Modified from: Cook Ch.E, Hegedus EJ. Orthopedic Physical Examination Tests: An Evidence-Based Approach (2nd Edition). Pearson Education Inc ., 2013 [40]

Number of positive tests	Sensitivity	Specificity	+LR	-LR
Two positive tests	98	14	1.1	0.14
Three positive tests	98	54	2.1	0.04
Four positive tests	77	83	4.6	0.28
Five positive tests	18	95	18.3	0.83

Building the nomogram representing the difference in pre-test probability (34% in this study) and post-test probability (CPR), the same author showed a 90% post-test probability to have CTS if five tests are positive; the probability dropped to 70% with four out of five tests positive. In fact, the CPR proposed by Wainner resulted in post-test probability changes of up to 56%. Furthermore, the interrater reliability was acceptable for all but two clinical examination items. (Tinel's B and the abductor pollicis brevis muscle test).

Graham et al. [80] developed a list of six clinical criteria (CTS-6) for the diagnosis of CTS, which were validated by statistical analysis after evaluation by panels of experts. These criteria are:

1 Numbness and tingling in the median nerve distribution,
2 Nocturnal numbness,
3 Weakness and/or atrophy of the thenar musculature,
4 Tinel's sign,
5 Phalen's test,
6 Loss of 2-point discrimination.

The six criteria had a statistically significant probability of being associated with a consensus diagnosis of CTS by the panel of physicians.

Hems [81] proposed a score system based on some symptoms and clinical signs, including Tinel's test, Phalen's test, and altered sensation. Points were attributed as follows: less than 60 years old =2 points; nocturnal pain =2 points; paresthesia =2 points, flick sign =2 points; improvement with splinting =1 point, clumsiness =1 point; positive Tinel's =2 points; positive Phalen's =1 point; hypasthesia =2 points; thenar eminence atrophy =2 points. A questionnaire threshold score equal to six points was selected for the diagnosis of CTS. When compared with NCS results, higher scores (at least 8 points) demonstrated specificity=67% and sensitivity=82% (see Table 11).

Table 11. Diagnostic accuracy of the Hems Score System. Modified from: Cook Ch.E, Hegedus EJ. Orthopedic Physical Examination Tests: An Evidence-Based Approach (2nd Edition). Pearson Education Inc., 2013 [40]

Score	Sensitivity	Specificity	+LR	-LR
6 points	92	61	2.36	0.13
7 points	82	67	2.48	0.27
8 points	70	72	2.5	0.42
6 symptoms	71	61	1.82	0.48

Finally, Amirfeyz et al. [73] proposed another combination of clinical tests: the tourniquet test, the carpal compression test and Phalen's test. Each of these tests significantly added value to the diagnosis: providing all three were positive, the area under the ROC curve was 0.98. However, we have observed that although combining some positive tests increases the likelihood of the diagnosis, negative or missing values confound its practical application.

Conclusion

The reliability and diagnostic accuracy of various tests commonly used in CTS appear discordant. Clinical tests should not be used as stand-alone tests, as they represent only a part of the clinical reasoning process, which also includes the history, neurological exam and nerve conduction testing. Insufficient uniformity in testing protocols makes comparing test results difficult. No single clinical test has been accepted as sufficient to identify this disorder, however the consideration of the severity of CTS might help interpret tests results. In fact, the sensitivity and specificity of a test could change at different stages of CTS. Furthermore, to evaluate the results of a study, an analysis of the cumulative effects of several tests performed on the same subject should be conducted.

To make the correct diagnosis, it is advisable to use a cluster of tests rather than a single test. The development of "clinical prediction rules" may be one of the most interesting perspectives for CTS diagnosis. Furthermore, diagnostic confirmation via a nerve conduction study would be appropriate.

References

[1]   Atroshi I, Gummersson C, Johnsson R, Ornstein E, Ranstam J, Ingmar R. Prevalence of carpal tunnel syndrome in a general population. *JAMA* 1999;282:153-8.

[2]   Rempel D, Evanoff B, Amadio P et al. Consensus criteria for the classification of carpal tunnel syndrome in epidemiologic studies. *American Journal of Public Health* 1998; 88:1447-1451.

[3]   Bland JD, Rudolfer SM- Clinical surveillance of carpal tunnel syndrome in two areas of the United Kingdom, 1991-2001 *J Neurol Neurosurg Psychiatry* 2003;74(12):1674-9.

[4]   De Krom MC, Knipschild PG, Kester AD, Thijs CT, Boekkooi PF, Spaans F. Carpal tunnel syndrome: prevalence in the general population. *J Clin Epidemiol* 1992;45(4):373-6.

[5]   Mondelli M, Giannini F, Giacchi M. Carpal tunnel syndrome incidence in a general population. *Neurology* 2002;58(2):289-94.

[6]   Phalen GS. The carpal-tunnel syndrome. Seventeen years' experience in diagnosis and treatment of six hundred fifty-four hands. *J Bone Joint Surg Am* 1966;48(2):211-28.

[7]   Stevens JC, Sun S, Beard CM, O'Fallon WM, Kurland LT. Carpal tunnel syndrome in Rochester, Minnesota, 1961 to 1980. *Neurology* 1988;38(1):134-8.

[8]   Tanaka S, Wild DK, Seligman PJ, Behrens V, Cameron L, Putz-Anderson V. The US prevalence of self-reported carpal tunnel syndrome *Am J Public Health* 1994;84(11):1846-8.

[9]   Hagberg M, Morgenster H, Kelsh M. Impact of occupation and job tasks on the prevalence of carpal tunnel syndrome. *Scad J Env Health*. 1992;18:337-345.

[10]   Glowacki KA, Breen CJ, Sachar K, Weiss AP. Electrodiagnostic testing and carpal tunnel release outcome. *The Journal of Hand Surgery* (Am) 1996;21(1):117-21.

[11]   Redmond MD, Rinver MH. False positive electrodiagnostic tests in carpal tunnel syndrome. *Muscle Nerve* 1988; 11:511–518.

[12] Homan MM, Franzblau A, Werner RA, Albers JW, Armstrong TJ, Bromberg MB. Agreement between symptom surveys, physical examination procedures and electrodiagnostic findings for the carpal tunnel syndrome. *Scand J Work Environ Health* 1999;25(2):1 15- 124.

[13] Violante FS, Bonfiglioli R, Isolani L, Raffi GB. Levels of agreement of nerve conduction studies and symptoms in workers at risk of carpal tunnel syndrome. *International Archives of Occupational and Environmental Health* 2004;77(8):552-8.

[14] American Association of Electrodiagnostic Medicine (AAEM), American Academy of Neurology, American Academy of Physical Medicine and Rehabilitation. Practice parameter for electrodiagnostic studies in carpal tunnel syndrome: summary statement. *Muscle Nerve* 2002;25:918-922.

[15] Jablecki CK, Andary MT, So YT, Wilkins DE, Williams FH. Literature review of the usefulness of nerve conduction studies and electromyography for the evaluation of patients with carpal tunnel syndrome. AAEM Quality Assurance Committee. *Muscle Nerve* 1993; 16(12):1392-414.

[16] Jablecki CK, Andary MT, Floeter MK, Miller RG, Quartly CA, Vennix MJ, Wilson JR; Practice parameter: Electrodiagnostic studies in carpal tunnel syndrome. *Report of the American Association of Electrodiagnostic Medicine, American Academy of Neurology, and the American Academy of Physical Medicine and Rehabilitation. Neurology.* 2002 Jun 11;58(11):1589-92.

[17] Kendall, D.: Aetiology, diagnosis and treatment of paraesthesiae in the hands. *British Med J* 1960;2:1633-1640.

[18] Yamaguchi DM, Lipscomb PR, Soule EH. Carpal Tunnel Syndrome. *Minn Med* 1965;48:22-33.

[19] Kongsholm J, Olerud C. *Carpal Tunnel Pressure in the Acute Phase After Colles' Fracture Arch Orthop Trauma Surg.* 1986;105:183-186.

[20] Kobayashi S, Baba H, Uchida K, Shimada S, Negoro K, Takeno K, Yayama T, Yamada S, Yoshizawa H. Localization and changes of intraneural inflammatory cytokines and inducible-nitric oxide induced by mechanical compression. *J Orthop Res.* 2005;23(4):771-8.

[21] Rempel DM, Diao E. Entrapment neuropathies: pathophysiology and pathogenesis. *J Electromyogr Kinesiol.* 2004 Feb;14(1):71-5.

[22] Rosenbaum RB. The role of imaging in the diagnosis of carpal tunnel syndrome. *Invest Radiol.* 1993;28(11):1059-62.

[23] Mackinnon SE, Novak CB. Clinical commentary: pathogenesis of cumulative trauma disorder. *J Hand Surg Am*. 1994;19(5):873-83.

[24] Colombini D, Occhipinti E, Cairoli S, Bettevi N, Menoni O, Ricci MG, Sferra C, Galletta A, Berlingò E, Draicchio F, Palmi S, Papale A, Di Loreto G. Barbieri PG, Niarinellamartineli I, Venturi E, De Vito G, Grieco A. Le affezioni muscoloscheletriche degli arti superiori e inferiori come patologie professionali; quali e a quali condizioni. Documento di consenso di un gruppo di lavoro nazionale. *Med Lav* 2003;94(3):312–329.

[25] Wainner RS, Fritz J, Irrgang J, Delitto A, Allison S, Boninger ML. Development of a clinical prediction rule for the diagnosis of carpal tunnel syndrome. *Arch Phys Med Rehabil* 2005;86:609-18.

[26] Buch-Jaeger N, Foucher G. Correlation of clinical signs with nerve conduction tests in the diagnosis of carpal tunnel syndrome. *J Hand Surg* [Br] 1994;19(6):720-4.

[27] Gupta SK, Benstead TJ. Symptoms experienced by patients with carpal tunnel syndrome. *Can J Neurol Sci*. 1997;24(4):338-42.

[28] Szabo RM, Slater RR, Jr., Farver TB, Stanton DB, Sharman WK. The value of diagnostic testing in carpal tunnel syndrome. *J Hand Surg [Am]* 1999;24(4):704-14.

[29] Katz JN, Stirrat CR, Larson MG, Fossel AH, Eaton HM, Liang MH. A self-administered hand symptom diagram for the diagnosis and epidemiologic study of carpal tunnel syndrome. *J Rheumatol* 1990;17(11):1495-8.

[30] D'Arcy CA, McGee S. Does this patient have carpal tunnel syndrome? *JAMA* 2000;283:3110–3117.

[31] Priganc VW, Henry SM. The relationship among five common carpal tunnel syndrome tests and the severity of carpal tunnel syndrome. *J Hand Ther*. 2003;16(3):225-36.

[32] Di Leo G., Vanti C. *Carpal tunnel syndrome – A review of the literature*. Scienza Riabilitativa 2010; 12(1): 16-27.

[33] Kuhlman KA, Hennessey WJ. Sensitivity and specificity of carpal tunnel syndrome signs. *Am J Phys Med Rehabil* 1997;76(6):451-7.

[34] Radecki P. A gender specific wrist ratio and the likelihood of a median nerve abnormality at the carpal tunnel. *Am J Phys Med Rehabil*. 1994;73(3):157-62.

[35] Omerr G.E. Jr, Spinne M. *Management of Peripheral Nerve Problems*. Philadelphia, WB Saunders, 1980.

[36] MacDermid JC, Doherty T. Clinical and Electrodiagnostic testing of Carpal Tunnel Syndrome: A Narrative Review. *The Journal of Orthopaedic and Sports Physical Therapy* 2004;34(10):565-588.

[37] Massy-Westropp N, Grimmer K, Bain G. A systematic review of the clinical diagnostic tests for carpal tunnel syndrome. *J Hand Surg Am.* 2000;25(1):120-7.

[38] Gelberman RH, Rydevik BL, Pess GM, Szabo RM, Lundborg G. Carpal tunnel syndrome. A scientific basis for clinical care. *Orthop Clin North Am.* 1988;19(1):115-24.

[39] Aroori S, Spence RAJ. Carpal tunnel syndrome. *Ulster Med J* 2008;77(1):6-17.

[40] Cook Ch.E, Hegedus EJ. *Orthopedic Physical Examination Tests: An Evidence-Based Approach* (2nd Edition). Pearson Education Inc, 2013.

[41] Kuschner SH, Ebramzadeh E, Johnson D, Brien WW, Sherman R. Tinel's sign and Phalen's test in carpal tunnel syndrome. *Orthopedics* 1992;15(11):1297-302.

[42] Mondelli M, Passero S, Giannini F. Provocative tests in different stages of carpal tunnel syndrome. *Clin Neurol Neurosurg* 2001;103(3):178-83.

[43] Valdes K, LaStayo P. The value of provocative tests for the wrist and elbow: A literature review. *J Hand Ther* 2013;26(1):32-42.

[44] Phalen GS, Kendrick JI. Compression neuropathy of the median nerve in the carpal tunnel. *J Am Med Assoc.* 1957; 164(5):524-30.

[45] De Krom MC, Knipshild PG, Kester AD, Spaans F. Efficacy of provocative tests for diagnosis of carpal tunnel syndrome. *Lancet* 1990;17(335):393-395.

[46] Williams TM, Mackinnon SE, Novak CB, McCabe S, Kelly L. Verification of the pressure provocative test in carpal tunnel syndrome. *Ann Plast Surg.* 1992;29(1):8-11.

[47] Tetro, Evanoff, Hollstien, Gelberman; A new provocative test for carpal tunnel syndrome. Assessment of wrist flexion and nerve compression. *J Bone Joint Surgery British* 1998;80(3):493–498.

[48] Nee B, Butler D. Management of peripheral neuropathic pain: Integrating neurobiology, neurodynamic and clinical evidence. *Phys Ther Sport* 2006; 36-49.

[49] Shacklock M. *Clinical Neurodynamics: A New System of Musculoskeletal Treatment.* Elsevier 2005.

[50] Vanti C, Bonfiglioli R, Calabrese M, Marinelli F, Guccione A, Violante FS, Pillastrini P. Upper Limb Neurodynamic Test 1 and symptoms

reproduction in carpal tunnel syndrome. *A validity Study. Man Ther.* 2011;16(3): 258-63.

[51] Kleinrensink GJ, Stoeckart R, Mulder PG, et al. Upper Limb Neurodynamic Tests as tools in the diagnosis of nerve and plexus lesions. Anatomical and biomechanical aspects. *Clin Biomech* (Bristol, Avon) 2000;15:9-14.

[52] Coppieters MW, Hough AD, Dilley A. Different nerve-gliding exercises induce different magnitudes of median nerve longitudinal excursion: An in vivo study using dynamic ultrasound imaging. *JOSPT* 2009;39(3):164-171.

[53] Vanti C, Conteddu L, Guccione A, Morsillo F, Parazza S, Viti C, Pillastrini P. The Upper Limb Neurodynamic Test 1: intra- and intertester reliability and the effect of several repetitions on pain and resistance. *J Manipulative Physiol Ther.* 2010;33(4):292-9.

[54] Butler DS. *The sensitive nervous system.* Adelaide, Unley: Noigroup Publication; 2000.

[55] Vanti C, Bonfiglioli R, Calabrese M, Marinelli F, Violante FS, Pillastrini P. Relationship between interpretation and accuracy of the Upper Limb Neurodynamic Test 1 in carpal tunnel syndrome. *J Manipulative Physiol Ther.* 2012;35(1):54-63.

[56] Coppieters MW, Alshami AM, Hodges PW. An Experimental Pain Model to Investigate the Specificity of the Neurodynamic test for the Median Nerve in the Differential Diagnosis of Hand Symptoms. *Arch Phys Med Rehabil* 2006;87:1412-1417.

[57] Nee RJ, Jull GA, Vicenzino B, Coppieters MW. The validity of upper-limb neurodynamic tests for detecting peripheral neuropathic pain. *JOSPT* 2012;42(5):413-24.

[58] Coppieters M, Stappaerts K, Janssens K, Jull G. Reliability of detecting 'onset of pain' and 'submaximal pain' during neural provocation testing for the upper quadrant. *Physiother Res Int* 2002;7(3):146-156.

[59] Edgar D, Jull G, Sutton S. The relationship between upper trapezius muscle length and upper quadrant neural tissue extensibility. *Aust J Physiother* 1994;40(2):99-103.

[60] Heide van der B, Allison GT, Zusman M. Pain and muscular responses to a neural tissue provocation test in the upper limb. *Man Ther* 2001;6(3):154-62.

[61] Reisch R, Williams K, Nee RJ, Rutt RA. ULNT2- Median Nerve Bias: Examiner Reliability and Sensory Responses in Asymptomatic Subjects. *The Journal of Manual and Manipulative Therapy* 2005;13(1):44-55.

[62] Schmid AB, Brunner F, Luomajoki H et al. Reliability of clinical tests to evaluate nerve function and mechanosensitivity of the upper limb peripheral nervous system. *BMC Musculoskelet Disord* 2009;21:10:11.

[63] Selvaratnam PJ, Matyas TA, Glasgow EF. Noninvasive discrimination of brachial plexus involvement in upper limb pain. *Spine* 1994;19(1):26-33.

[64] Wainner RS, Fritz JM, Irrgang JJ, Boninger ML, Delitto A, Allison S. Reliability and Diagnostic Accuracy of the Clinical Examination and Patient Self-Report Measures for Cervical Radiculopathy. *Spine* 2003;28(1):52-62.

[65] Walsh M. Upper limb neural tension testing and mobilization. Fact, Fiction, and a Practical Approach. *J Hand Ther* 2005;18(2):241-58.

[66] Vanti C., Conteddu L., Guccione A., Morsillo F., Parazza S., Viti C., Pillastrini P. The Upper Limb Neurodynamic Test 1: intra- and inter-tester reliability and the effect of several repetitions on Pain and Resistance. *Journal of Manipulative and Physiological Therapeutics* 2010; 33(4): 292-9.

[67] Coveney B, Trott P, Grimmer K, Bell A, Hall, Shacklock M. The upper limb tension test in a group of subject with a clinical presentation of carpal tunnel syndrome. In: *Proceedings of the Manipulative Physiotherapists' Association of Australia, Melbourne*; 1997:31-33.

[68] Mahmud MAI, Merlo ARC, Gomes I, Becker J, Nora DB. Relationship between adverse neural tension and nerve conduction studies in patients with symptoms of the carpal tunnel syndrome. *Arq Neuropsiquiatr* 2006; 64(2-A):277-282.

[69] LaBan MM, Friedman NA, Zemenick GA. 'Tethered' median nerve stress test in chronic carpal tunnel syndrome. *Arch Phys Med Rehabil* 1986;67(11):803-804.

[70] Kaul MP, Pagel KJ, Dryden JD. Lack of predictive power of the "tethered" median stress test in suspected carpal tunnel syndrome. *Arch Phys Med Rehabil* 2000;81(3):348-50.

[71] Ahn DS. Hand elevation: a new test for carpal tunnel syndrome. *Ann Plast Surg.* 2001;46(2):120-4.

[72] Amirfeyz R, Gozzard C, Leslie IJ. Hand elevation test for assessment of carpal tunnel syndrome. *J Hand Surg Br.* 2005;30(4):361-4.

[73] Amirfeyz R, Clark D, Parsons B, Melotti R, Bhatia R, Leslie I, Bannister G. Clinical tests for carpal tunnel syndrome in contemporary Practice. *Arch Orthop Trauma Surg* 2010:e-pub ahead of print.

[74] Karl AI, Carney ML, Kaul MP. The lumbrical provocation test in subjects with median inclusive paresthesia. *Arch Phys Med Rehabil.* 2001;82(7):935-7.

[75] Yii NW, Elliot D. A study of the dynamic relationship of the lumbrical muscles and the carpal tunnel. *J Hand Surg Br.* 1994;19(4):439-43.

[76] Golding DN, Rose DM, Selvarajah K. Clinical tests for carpal tunnel syndrome: an evaluation. *Br J Rheumatol* 1986;25(4):388-90.

[77] Gellman H, Gelderman RH, Tam AM, Botte MG. Carpal tunnel syndrome. An evaluation of the provocative diagnostic test. *J Bone Joint Surg Am* 1986; 68:735-7.

[78] Descatha A, Dale AM, Franzblau A, Coomes J, Evanoff B. Diagnostic strategies using physical examination are minimally useful in defining carpal tunnel syndrome in population-based research studies. *Occupational and Environmental Medicine* 2010;67:133-135.

[79] Bickel KD. Carpal tunnel syndrome. J Hand Surg Am. 2010;35(1):147-52.

[80] Graham B, Regehr G, Naglie G, Wright JG. Development and validation of diagnostic criteria for carpal tunnel syndrome. *J Hand Surg* 2006;31A:919–924.

[81] Hems TE, Miller R, Massraf A, Green J. Assessment of a diagnostic questionnaire and protocol for management of carpal tunnel syndrome. *J Han Surg Eur* Vol. 2009;34(5):665-70.

[82] Gunnarsson LG, Amilon A, Hellstrand P, Leissner P, Philipson L. The diagnosis of carpal tunnel syndrome. Sensitivity and specificity of some clinical and electrophysiological tests. *Journal of Hand Surgery* 1997;22B: 34–37.

[83] Katz JN, Stirrat CR. A self-administered hand diagram for the diagnosis of carpal tunnel syndrome. *J Hand Surg Am.* 1990;15(2):360-3.

[84] Katz JN, Larson MG, Sabra A, Krarup C, Stirrat CR, Sethi R, Eaton HM, Fossel AH, Liang MH. The carpal tunnel syndrome: diagnostic utility of the history and physical examination findings. *Ann Intern Med.* 1990;112(5):321-7.

[85] O'Gradaigh D, Merry P. A diagnostic algorithm for carpal tunnel syndrome based on Bayes's theorem. Rheumatology (Oxford). 2000;39(9):1040-1.

[86] Borg K, Lindblom U. Increase of vibration threshold during wrist flexion in patients with carpal tunnel syndrome. *Pain* 1986;26(2):211-9.

[87] Brüske J, Bednarski M, Niedźwiedź Z, Zyluk A, Grzeszewski S. The usefulness of the Phalen test and the Hoffmann-Tinel sign in the

diagnosis of carpal tunnel syndrome. *Acta Orthop Belg*. 2002;68(2):141-5.

[88]   Cheng CJ, Mackinnon-Patterson B, Beck JL, Mackinnon SE. Scratch collapse test for evaluation of carpal and cubital tunnel syndrome. *J Hand Surg Am*. 2008;33: 1518e1524.

[89]   Durkan JA. A new diagnostic test for carpal tunnel syndrome. *J Bone Joint Surg* 1991;73: 535-8.

[90]   Gelmers HJ. The significance of Tinel's sign in the diagnosis of carpal tunnel syndrome. *Acta Neurochir* (Wien). 1979;49(3-4):255-8.

[91]   Gerr F, Letz R. The sensitivity and specificity of tests for carpal tunnel syndrome vary with the comparison subjects. *J Hand Surg Br*. 1998;23(2):151-5.

[92]   Gonzalez Del Pino J, Delgado-Martinez AD, Gonzalez I, Lovic A. Value of the carpal compression test in the diagnosis of carpal tunnel syndrome. *J Hand Surg* 1997;22B:38–41.

[93]   Hansen PA, Micklesen P, Robinson LR: Clinical utility of the flick maneuver in diagnosing carpal tunnel syndrome. *Am J Phys Med Rehabil* 2004;83:363–367.

[94]   Heller L, Ring H, Costeff H, Solzi P. Evaluation of Tinel's and Phalen's signs in diagnosis of the carpal tunnel syndrome. *Eur. Neurol.* 1986;25(1):40-2.

[95]   LaJoie AS, McCabe SJ, Thomas B, Edgell SE. Determining the sensitivity and specificity of common diagnostic tests for carpal tunnel syndrome using latent class analysis. *Plast Reconstr Surg.* 2005;116:502e507.

[96]   El Miedany Y, Ashour S, Youssef S, Mehanna A, Meky FA. Clinical diagnosis of carpal tunnel syndrome: old tests-new concepts. *Joint Bone Spine.* 2008;75(4):451-7.

[97]   Seror P. Tinel's sign in the diagnosis of carpal tunnel syndrome. *J Hand Surg Br.* 1987;12(3):364-5.

[98]   Stewart JD, Eisen A. Tinel's sign and the carpal tunnel syndrome. *Br Med J.* 1978;2(6145):1125-6.

[99]   Wainner RS, Boninger ML, Balu G, Burdett R, Helkowski W. Durkan gauge and carpal compression test: accuracy and diagnostic test properties. *J Orthop Sports Phys Ther.* 2000 Nov;30(11):676-82.

[100]   Walters C, Rice V. An evaluation of provocative testing in the diagnosis of carpal tunnel syndrome. *Mil Med.* 2002;167(8):647-52.

[101]   Boland RA, Kiernan MC. Assessing the accuracy of a combination of clinical tests for identifying carpal tunnel syndrome. *J Clin Neurosci.*

2009;16(7):929-33Burke FD. Carpal tunnel syndrome. *Ann R Coll Surg Engl.* 2007;89(1):88-9.

[103] De Smet L, Steenwerckx A, Van den Bogaert G, Cnudde P, Fabry G. Value of clinical provocative tests in carpal tunnel syndrome. *Acta Orthop Belg* 1995;61(3):177-82.

[104] Durkan JA. The carpal-compression test. An instrumented device for diagnosing carpal tunnel syndrome. *Orthop Rev.* 1994;23(6):522-5.

[105] Fertl E, Wöber C, Zeitlhofer J. The serial use of two provocative tests in the clinical diagnosis of carpal tunel syndrome. *Acta Neurol Scand.*1998;98(5):328-32.

[106] *Tekeoglu I, Dogan A, Demir G, Dolar.* The pneumatic compression test and modified pneumatic compression test in the diagnosis of carpal tunnel syndrome. *E. Journal of Hand Surgery, European Vol 2007 32: 697*

[107] Pryse-Phillips WE. Validation of a diagnostic sign in carpal tunnel syndrome. *J Neurol Neurosurg Psychiatry.* 1984;47(8):870-2.

In: Carpal Tunnel Syndrome
Editor: Morton Ledford

ISBN: 978-1-63321-142-1
© 2014 Nova Science Publishers, Inc.

Chapter 5

Patient Evaluation Measure and Michigan Hand Outcome Measure

Wasim S. Khan, Ph.D.[1,*] *and Mark A. Ravenscroft, FRCS*[2]

[1]University College London Institute of Orthopaedics and Musculoskeletal Sciences, Royal National Orthopaedic Hospital, Stanmore, London, UK
[2]Department of Trauma and Orthopaedics, Stockport NHS Foundation Trust, Stepping Hill Hospital, Stockport, UK

Abstract

Injuries and disease commonly affect the hand and these can significantly affect the ability of an individual to perform activities of daily living. The use of regional outcome measures or scoring systems is important as it allows comparison between these injuries and disease, and allows clinicians to assess progression and the effects of different treatment modalities. A patient-completed questionnaire is efficient in terms of time and resources, and allows the assessment of outcome without the need to attend an outpatient clinic. It is important that the scoring system allows satisfactory regional outcome measurements specific for the hand.

---

* Corresponding author: Mr. Wasim S. Khan, Academic Clinical Fellow, University College London Institute of Orthopaedics and Musculoskeletal Science, Royal National Orthopaedic Hospital, Stanmore, London, HA7 4LP, UK. Telephone number: +44 (0) 7971 190720, Fax number: +44 (0) 20 8570 3864, E-mail address: wasimkhan@doctors.org.uk.

The validity, reliability, responsiveness and bias are used for the assessment of various questionnaires. There are also many practical issues concerning the use of questionnaires including feasibility of use for the patient and the clinician.

The Patient Evaluation Measure (PEM) questionnaire, and the Michigan Hand Outcome (MHO) questionnaire are a few of the region-specific outcome measures commonly used for the hand, and are patient-completed questionnaires. They are frequently used to assess self-reported patient outcome in orthopaedics, rheumatology and neurology. In this paper, the validity, reliability, responsiveness and bias of these two questionnaires used for the assessment of the hand will be discussed.

Patient Evaluation Measure Questionnaire

The Patient Evaluation Measure (PEM) questionnaire was developed in the United Kingdom in 1995 by Macey et al. and assesses patient satisfaction with treatment, general hand functioning and activities of daily living. Unlike the Disabilities of the Arm, Shoulder and Hand (DASH) and Michigan Hand Outcome (MHO) questionnaires, it has not formally been psychometrically evaluated.

There are only a few studies that have statistically analysed the questionnaire. Dias et al. (2001) studied the reliability, validity, responsiveness and bias of the questionnaire (Table 1), and found it to be reliable, valid, responsive and free from bias. They studied 80 patients with acute scaphoid fractures at two, eight, twelve, twenty-six and fifty-two weeks following injury. The patients had a mean age of 29.7 years (SD 10.1 years). Patients with pre-existing wrist or hand disorders were excluded from the study. The patients were assessed at each visit where a history was taken and the patient examined. The patients were questioned about pain and swelling, the hand was examined for tenderness, range of wrist movements were measured using a goniometer, grip strength was measured using a dynamometer, and patients were asked to complete the PEM questionnaire.

The PEM questionnaire has a simple, uncluttered and easy to follow layout.

Questions are short and simple, and are in a visual analogue form, and the patients only have to read the question, and not the description of the interval answers.

The questions can be answered on a seven-interval visual analogue scale. The questionnaire is easy to enter into a database and to analyse.

Table 1. Patient Evaluation Measure (PEM) questionnaire

Please put a circle around the number that is the closest to the way you feel about how things have been for you. There are no right or wrong answers.							
Part one- treatment							
1. Throughout my treatment I have seen the same doctor	1	2	3	4	5	6	7
	Every time						Not all the time
2. When the doctor saw me, he or she knew about my case	1	2	3	4	5	6	7
	Very well						Not at all
3. When I was with the doctor, he or she gave me the chance to talk	1	2	3	4	5	6	7
	As much as I wanted						Not at all
4. When I did talk to the doctor, he or she listened and understood me	1	2	3	4	5	6	7
	Very much						Not at all
5. I was given information about my treatment and progress	1	2	3	4	5	6	7
	All that I wanted						Not at all
Part two- how is your hand now? Hand health profile							
1. The feeling in my hand is now	1	2	3	4	5	6	7
	Normal						Absent
2. When my hand is cold and/or damp, my hand is now	1	2	3	4	5	6	7
	Non-existent						Unbearable

Table 1. (Continued)

Please put a circle around the number that is the closest to the way you feel about how things have been for you. There are no right or wrong answers.								
Part two- how is your hand now? Hand health profile								
3. Most of the time, the pain in my hand is now	1	2	3	4	5	6	7	
	Non-existent						Unbearable	
4. The duration my pain is present is	1	2	3	4	5	6	7	
	Never						All the time	
5. When I try to use my hand for fiddly things, it is now	1	2	3	4	5	6	7	
	Skilful						Clumsy	
6. Generally when I move my hand it is	1	2	3	4	5	6	7	
	Flexible						Stiff	
7. The grip in my hand is now	1	2	3	4	5	6	7	
	Strong						Weak	
8. For everyday activities, my hand is now	1	2	3	4	5	6	7	
	No problem						Useless	
9. For my work, my hand is now	1	2	3	4	5	6	7	
	No problem						Useless	
10. When I look at the appearance of my hand now, I feel	1	2	3	4	5	6	7	
	Unconcerned						Embarrassed and self-conscious	
11. Generally when I think about my hand I feel	1	2	3	4	5	6	7	
	Unconcerned						Very upset	

Please put a circle around the number that is the closest to the way you feel about how things have been for you. There are no right or wrong answers.							
Part three- overall assessment							
1. Generally, my treatment at the hospital has been	1	2	3	4	5	6	7
	Very satisfactory						Very unsatisfactory
2. Generally, my hand is now	1	2	3	4	5	6	7
	Very satisfactory						Very unsatisfactory
3. Bearing in mind my original injury and condition, I feel my hand is now	1	2	3	4	5	6	7
	Better than I expected						Worse than I expected

The questionnaire included three sections including a five question section assessing patients' view of treatment, and three question section assessing patients' overall assessment. There was an eleven question section assessing the hand health profile and included an added question on duration of pain that was absent in the original questionnaire. The PEM questionnaire score was calculated by adding the response to each question from sections two and three, and expressing the sum as a percentage of the maximum possible score.

The validity was assessed by determining how well responses to each question of the questionnaire and the total PEM questionnaire score, correlated with subjective and objective measures of function including pain, tenderness, swelling, wrist movements and grip strength.

The study showed that the PEM was highly valid since it correlated well with other measures commonly used in the assessments of the function of the wrist and hand. Each individual question and the total PEM questionnaire score correlated well with the pain, tenderness, swelling, range of movement and grip strength. They established that the questions in the PEM questionnaire are highly internally consistent. The questions address different facets of the symptoms, function and cosmesis of the hand. The face validity of the questionnaire appears sound; it includes questions not usually included in the assessment of patients e.g. 'When I look at the appearance of my hand now, I feel: unconcerned......... embarrassed and self-conscious' and 'Generally, when I think about my hand I feel: unconcerned....... very upset'.

The reliability was assessed by measuring the internal consistency of the eleven questions in the hand health profile section and the three questions in the overall assessment section. They measured the correlation of each question with the others and generated Cronbach's alpha. The correlations of some of the questions e.g. 'When I try to use my hand for fiddly things, it is now: skilful......... clumsy', 'The grip in my hand is now: strong......... weak' and 'Generally, my hand is now: very satisfactory......... very unsatisfactory' with the rest of the scale was high at 0.83, 0.84 and 0.84, respectively. The correlations of some questions e.g. 'When I look at the appearance of my hand now, I feel: unconcerned.......... embarrassed and self-conscious', 'Generally when I think about my hand I feel: unconcerned.......... very upset' and 'Generally, my treatment at the hospital has been: very satisfactory.......... very unsatisfactory' with the rest of the scale was particularly low at 0.36, 0.43 and 0.34 respectively.

The questionnaire was considered to be internally consistent if Cronbach's alpha was between 0.7 and 0.9. The Cronbach's alpha, calculating from these correlations was found to be 0.9, and suggested internal consistency. A very high internal consistency of >0.9 suggests that there is some redundancy with questions are measuring the same aspect twice. There was overall correlation across visits and for each visit. Cronbach's alpha at weeks 2, 8, 12, 26 and 52, were 0.874, 0.905, 0.939, 0.912 and 0.911 respectively. The overall value over time was 0.932 because of the added effect of the correlation due to changes in the group mean score over time. If a question disproportionately contributes to the internal consistency, then deleting it will result in a fall in Cronbach's alpha. If a question does not disproportionately contribute to the internal consistency, then deleting it will cause the Cronbach's alpha will rise. In the study, the Cronbach's alpha remained close to the 0.9, suggesting that each question contributed to the overall score and the PEM questionnaire is reliable. The degree of contribution of each question was studied by measuring the corrected Cronbach's alpha value after excluding that particular item.

To assess responsiveness, the changes between visits in the PEM questionnaire score and the pain, tenderness, swelling, wrist movement and grip strength were assessed.

Changes in the PEM questionnaire score were correlated with changes in each of the other variables. Responsiveness was measured by calculating the effect size and by assessing the standardised response mean.

Responsiveness was assessed by looking at the correlation between the variation in the questionnaire to changes in pain, tenderness, swelling, range of movement and grip strength.

Pain and grip strength correlated significantly (p < 0.001) with changes in the PEM questionnaire score between the second and eighth weeks. Tenderness, range of movement and grip strength correlated significantly (p < 0.03) with changes in the PEM questionnaire score between the eighth and fifty second weeks. The effect size was calculated by dividing the mean of the change in the PEM questionnaire score between visits by the standard deviation of the baseline PEM questionnaire score. The effect size for the PEM questionnaire score was 1.12 and, as it was greater than 0.8, it was valuable. This effect size matched the effect sizes for swelling, tenderness, range of movement and grip strength at various stages between the second and fifty second weeks. The standardised response mean was calculated by dividing the mean of change in the PEM questionnaire score between visits at weeks 2 and 8 and between weeks 8 and 52 by the standard deviation of the change in PEM questionnaire score.

The standardised response mean was 1.46 and 1.47 between visits at weeks 2 and 8 and between weeks 8 and 52 respectively. These assessments suggested that the PEM questionnaire is highly responsive.

Bias was studied by measuring the variance of each PEM question and the PEM questionnaire score for assumed independent variables including gender, hand dominance, the side injured and injuries to the dominant hand. Age bias was studied by correlating age with the PEM questionnaire score. The effects of subject factors were tested in a repeated measures analysis of variance, incorporating a fixed effect for the visit and a random effect for the subject. The study showed no item bias for gender, dominance and side injured. There was significant correlation with age at 0.01, suggesting that older patients had a lower PEM questionnaire score. This finding may be due to a poorer outcome in older individuals, and this was supported by a regression analysis of age and grip strength (p= 0.002).

The study concluded that the PEM is internally consistent, highly valid and responsive. They showed that gender, age, handedness and side injured did not cause bias in the responses to the questions. One potential flaw in the methodology of this study was that at each visit, the patients were told what their questionnaire answers had been at their previous visit. This could have determined the subsequent responses but nevertheless was needed to avoid bias and would have improved the consistency for this visual analogue scale response.

In 2005, Hobby et al. studied the validity of the PEM questionnaire as an outcome measure in 24 patients with carpal tunnel syndrome before and three months after decompression.

The validity of the PEM questionnaire was compared with the DASH questionnaire and with objective hand function measurements including grip strength, static two-point discrimination and the nine-hole peg test.

The responsiveness of the PEM questionnaire following carpal tunnel decompression was also compared with that of the DASH questionnaire. There was a significant correlation between the PEM and DASH questionnaire scores, and between individual questions of the PEM questionnaire and the objective measurements. The PEM questionnaire showed a greater responsiveness to change than the DASH score with an effect size of 0.97 compared with 0.49.

In 2007, Forward et al. studied the validity and internal consistency of the PEM questionnaire in 200 patients with distal radius fracture. They assessed the patients six to forty-two years after injury using the PEM and DASH questionnaires and objective measures of outcome including grip and pinch strength and range of movement. They found highly significant correlations between the PEM and DASH questionnaires, and between the PEM questionnaire and objective measures. One drawback of the study is the use of PEM questionnaires completed for both the injured and uninjured wrist, and then used to calculate a comparative PEM score by subtracting the score of the uninjured wrist from that of the injured side, to eliminate the effect of co-existing disease. This score was found to more strongly correlate with outcome than the PEM score alone. The authors concluded that the PEM questionnaire was a valid method of assessing distal radial fracture outcome.

Michigan Hand Outcome Questionnaire

The Michigan Hand Outcome (MHO) questionnaire assesses hand function, activities of daily living, work performance, pain, aesthetics and satisfaction. The MHO questionnaire, like the DASH, was developed for use in North America. In 1998, Chung et al. developed the questionnaire (Table 2) after assessing outcome measures considered important by a panel of patients, hand therapists and hand surgeons. Chung et al. describe the development of the questionnaire including the initial psychometric testing, and assessment of the reliability and validity.

The authors used a literature search of pre-existing questionnaires to identify questions related to upper limb function and created a preliminary version of the MHO questionnaire. A panel of patients were also asked to produce relevant questions.

Table 2. Michigan Hand Outcome (MHO) questionnaire

Instructions: This survey asks for your views about your hands and your health. This information will help keep track of how you feel and how well you are able to do your usual activities. Answer *every* question by marking the answer as indicated. If you are unsure about how to answer a question, please give the best answer you can.

I. The following questions refer to the function of your hand(s)/wrist(s) *during the past week*. (Please circle I answer for each question.)

A. The following questions refer to your *right* hand/wrist.

	Very Good	Good	Fair	Poor	Very Poor
1. Overall, how well did your *right* hand work?	1	2	3	4	5
2. How well did your *right* fingers move?	1	2	3	4	5
3. How well did your *right* wrist move?	1	2	3	4	5
4. How was the strength in your *right* hand?	1	2	3	4	5
5. How was the sensation (feeling) in your *right* hand'?	1	2	3	4	5

B. The following questions refer to your *left* hand/wrist.

	Very Good	Good	Fair	Poor	Very Poor
1. Overall, how well did your *left* hand work?	1	2	3	4	5
2. How well did your *left* fingers move?	1	2	3	4	5
3. How well did your *left* wrist move?	1	2	3	4	5
4. How was the strength in your *left* hand?	1	2	3	4	5
5. How was the sensation (feeling) in your *left* hand'?	1	2	3	4	5

II. The following questions refer to the ability of your hand(s) to do certain tasks *during the past week*. (Please circle 1 answer for each question.)

A. How difficult was it for you to perform the following activities using your *right hand*?

	Not at All Difficult	A Little Difficult	Somewhat Difficult	Moderately Difficult	Very Difficult
1. Turn a door knob	1	2	3	4	5
2. Pick up a coin	1	2	3	4	5
3. Hold a glass of water	1	2	3	4	5
4. Turn a key in a lock	1	2	3	4	5
5. Hold a frying pan	1	2	3	4	5

Table 2. (Continued)

B. How difficult was it for you to perform the following activities using your *left hand?*					
	Not at All Difficult	A Little Difficult	Somewhat Difficult	Moderately Difficult	Very Difficult
1. Turn a door knob	1	2	3	4	5
2. Pick up a coin	1	2	3	4	5
3. Hold a glass of water	1	2	3	4	5
4. Turn a key in a lock	1	2	3	4	5
5. Hold a frying pan	1	2	3	4	5

C. How difficult was it for you to perform the following activities using *both of your hands?*					
	Not at All Difficult	A Little Difficult	Somewhat Difficult	Moderately Difficult	Very Difficult
1. Open a, jar	1	2	3	4	5
2. Button a shirt/blouse	1	2	3	4	5
3. Eat with a knife/fork	1	2	3	4	5
4. Carry a grocery bag	1	2	3	4	5
5. Wash dishes	1	2	3	4	5
6. Wash your hair	1	2	3	4	5
7. Tie shoelaces/knots	1	2	3	4	5

III. The following questions refer to how you did in your *normal work* (including both housework and school work) during the past *4 weeks.* (Please circle 1 answer for each question.)					
	Always	Often	Sometimes	Rarely	Never
1. How often were you unable to do your work because of problems with your hand(s)/wrist(s)?	1	2	3	4	5
2. How often did you have to shorten your work day because of problems with your hand(s)/ wrist(s)?	1	2	3	4	5
3. How often did you have to take it easy at your work because of problems with your hand(s)/wrist(s)?	1	2	3	4	5
4. How often did you accomplish less in your work because of problems with your hand(s)/wrist(s)?	1	2	3	4	5

III. The following questions refer to how you did in your *normal work* (including both housework and school work) during the past *4 weeks.* (Please circle 1 answer for each question.)

	Always	Often	Sometimes	Rarely	Never
5. How often did you take longer to do the tasks in your work because of problems with your hand(s)/wrist(s)?	1	2	3	4	5

IV. The following questions refer to how much *pain* you had in your hand(s)/wrist(s) *during the past week* (Please circle 1 answer for each question.)

1. How often did you have pain in your hand(s)/wrist(s)?	1. Always	2. Often	3. Sometimes	4. Rarely	5. Never

If you answered *never* to *question IV-1* above, please skip the following questions and go to the next section.

2. Please describe the pain you have in your hand(s)/wrist(s).	1. Very mild	2. Mild	3. Moderate	4. Severe	5. Very severe

	Always	Often	Sometimes	Rarely	Never
3. How often did the pain in your hand(s)/wrist(s) interfere with your sleep'?	1	2	3	4	5
4. How often did the pain in your hand(s)/wrist(s) interfere with your daily activities (such as eating or bathing)?	1	2	3	4	5
5. How often did the pain in your hand(s)/wrist(s) make you unhappy'?	1	2	3	4	5

V. A. The following questions refer to the appearance (look) of your *right* hand during the past week. (Please circle 1 answer for each question.)

	Strongly Agree	Agree	Neither Agree Nor Disagree	Disagree	Strongly Disagree
1. I was satisfied with the appearance (look) of my *right* hand.	1	2	3	4	5
2. The appearance (look) of my *right* hand sometimes made me uncomfortable in public.	1	2	3	4	5
3. The appearance (look) of my *right* hand made me depressed.	1	2	3	4	5

Table 2. (Continued)

V. A. The following questions refer to the appearance (look) of your *right* hand during the past week. (Please circle 1 answer for each question.)					
	Strongly Agree	*Agree*	*Neither Agree Nor Disagree*	*Disagree*	*Strongly Disagree*
4. The appearance (look) of my *right* hand interfered with my normal social activities	1	2	3	4	5

B. The following questions refer to the appearance (look) of your *left* hand during the past week. (Please circle 1 answer for each question.)					
	Strongly Agree	*Agree*	*Neither Agree Nor Disagree*	*Disagree*	*Strongly Disagree*
1. I was satisfied with the appearance (look) of my *left* hand.	1	2	3	4	5
2. The appearance (look) of my *left* hand sometimes made me uncomfortable in public.	1	2	3	4	5
3. The appearance (look) of my *left* hand made me depressed.	1	2	3	4	5
4. The appearance (look) of my *left* hand interfered with my normal social activities	1	2	3	4	5

VI. A. The following questions refer to your satisfaction with your *right* hand/wrist during the past week. (Please circle 1 answer for each question.)					
	Very Satisfied	*Somewhat Satisfied*	*Neither Satisfied Nor Dissatisfied*	*Somewhat Dissatisfied*	*Dissatisfied*
1. Overall function of your *right* hand	1	2	3	4	5
2. Motion of the fingers in your *right* Hand	1	2	3	4	5
3. Motion of your *right* wrist	1	2	3	4	5
4. Strength of your *right* hand	1	2	3	4	5
5. Pain level of your *right* hand	1	2	3	4	5

VI. A. The following questions refer to your satisfaction with your *right* hand/wrist during the past week. (Please circle 1 answer for each question.)					
	Very Satisfied	Somewhat Satisfied	Neither Satisfied Nor Dissatisfied	Somewhat Dissatisfied	Dissatisfied
6. Sensation (feeling) of your *right* Hand	1	2	3	4	5

B. The following questions refer to your satisfaction with your *left* hand/wrist during the past week. (Please circle 1 answer for each question.)					
	Very Satisfied	Somewhat Satisfied	Neither Satisfied Nor Dissatisfied	Somewhat Dissatisfied	Dissatisfied
1. Overall function of your *left* hand	1	2	3	4	5
2. Motion of the fingers in your *left* Hand	1	2	3	4	5
3. Motion of your *left* wrist	1	2	3	4	5
4. Strength of your *left* hand	1	2	3	4	5
5. Pain level of your *left* hand	1	2	3	4	5
6. Sensation (feeling) of your *left* hand	1	2	3	4	5

This resulted in 100 questions that were then evaluated by a panel of patients, hand therapists and hand surgeons. It was determined that the questions would fall into six domains: overall hand function, activities of daily living, pain, work performance, aesthetics and patient satisfaction with hand function.

The preliminary version of the MHO questionnaire was also evaluated by two psychometricians with experience in the designing of questionnaire, and redundant questions were eliminated and wordings modified. Factor analysis was used to further decrease the number of questions in the six domains to 37. Four domains, overall hand function, activities of daily living, aesthetics, and satisfaction with hand function, contain questions for both right and left hand to offset the confounding effect of hand dominance.

After the MHO questionnaire had been revised, it was pilot tested in 200 patients waiting for their first appointment at a hand clinic. The patients also completed a SF-12 questionnaire. To calculate the score, the responses to all questions were added and normalised to a scale from 0 to 100.

In the pain domain, a higher score indicates greater pain and a lower score indicates less pain.

In the remaining five domains, a higher score indicates better hand function and a lower score indicates poorer hand function. Validity and reliability were tested.

Content or face validity indicates whether the questionnaire appears logical to a group of experts. A panel of patients with hand disorders, hand therapists and hand surgeons evaluated the questionnaire for content validity.

Construct validity assesses the domains in the questionnaire to see if they perform as expected compared with other measures e.g. the SF-12.

To investigate the construct validity, the six domains were analysed for correlations with each other. The Spearman's rank correlation showed a high correlation among the five functional domains: overall hand function, activities of daily living, work performance, pain, and satisfaction with hand function. The aesthetics domain however showed a weaker correlation with the other scales with values ranging from -0.29 to 0.46. Only three of the domains in the MHO questionnaire were compared with the SF-12 questionnaire, and these were activities of daily living, work performance and pain. Although the pain domain had a substantial correlation with the pain question in the SF-12, the activities of daily living and work performance domains only had a moderate correlation.

To determine the domains that were significant predictors of physical function, all domains were regressed against the physical function component of the SF-12. The activities of daily living, overall hand function and aesthetics domains did not show a significant relation with physical function.

Reliability was evaluated using test-retest and internal consistency. For test-retest reliability, patients completed the questionnaire at their first appointment in the clinic and a week later at home. The scores for each domain were correlated for the first and the second time point using interclass correlation. Although they had an overall response rate of 99%, the test-retest reliability was only assessed in 22 patients. Intra-class correlation was used to assess test-retest reliability where a score of 1.0 suggests perfect correlation and a score of 0 suggests no correlation.

Test-retest analyses showed excellent correlation for the six domains and all domains except aesthetics had correlation scores over 0.85. The mean difference in the questionnaire scores between the time points was also measured to determine if the scores agreed, and showed excellent agreement suggesting good test-retest reliability. Again, this was only done in 22 patients.

Internal consistency measures the homogeneity of the questions that make up a domain and determine if the questions in the domain are highly correlated with each other.

A high inter-item correlation suggests that the questions in a domain are all measuring the same thing. Internal consistency is expressed by Cronbach's alpha that can range from 0 to 1.0, where 1.0 suggests perfect internal consistency and 0 suggests no internal consistency.

Generally, Cronbach's alpha values of greater than 0.80 in a domain are considered acceptable and values for the six domains ranged from 0.86-0.97 suggesting excellent internal consistency. The Cronbach's alphas were high in testing for internal consistency. High Cronbach's alphas could also indicate redundancy in the domains, and the authors suggested that efforts to develop a shorter version of the MHO questionnaire should be considered.

Although the authors state that the self-administered questionnaire could be completed in 10 minutes and that patients indicated that it was an acceptable length, our experience differs.

In 2004, Massy-Westropp et al. evaluated the validity and reliability of the of the MHO questionnaire for assessing disability in 62 patients with rheumatoid arthritis. Although the MHO provided patient and context-specific information, the Sequential Occupational Dexterity Assessment (SODA) questionnaire provided more impairment information that could readily be compared between patients.

The pain domain of the MHO questionnaire correlated well with the Australian Canadian Osteoarthritis Hand Index (AUSCAN) questionnaire (r=0.68). Seventeen patients also repeated the questionnaires within five days showing good reliability. The MHO questionnaire has the advantage that it provides information on both hands, and the authors state that clinicians should decide whether bilateral or unilateral hand function is of interest before choosing a questionnaire. The authors concluded that the MHO questionnaire is valid and reliable for assessment of hand disability in rheumatoid patients.

In 2008, Sambandam et al. studied the development, validity, reliability, responsiveness and limitations of six different carpal tunnel syndrome outcome measures including the Boston Carpal Tunnel Questionnaire (BCTQ), MHO questionnaire, DASH questionnaire, PEM questionnaire, clinical rating scale (Historical-Objective (Hi-Ob) scale) and Upper Extremity Functional Scale (UEFS).

They concluded that the BCTQ, MHO and PEM questionnaires had good validity, reliability and responsiveness both in the hands of the developers of the questionnaires, as well as independent researchers.

They also stated that the DASH questionnaire has a potential role in the assessment of carpal tunnel syndrome but requires more validation in exclusive carpal tunnel patients.

In 2008, Dias et al. studied the construct and criterion validity, reliability, and acceptability of the PEM, MHO and DASH questionnaires in 100 patients with different hand and wrist disorders.

They found that the internal consistency of all three questionnaires was very high suggesting some redundancy in questions.

They also found that all questionnaires were valid, reliable and reproducible for finger and wrist disorders with a high correlation between the domains.

They also studied ease of use using a questionnaire and found that the PEM was the easiest to understand and complete, taking the least time.

The values for the Manchester-Modified DASH (M2DASH), PEM and MHO questionnaires from 40 patients were plot against each other on scatter plots to determine the relationships between them (Khan et al., in press).

The M2 DASH and PEM scores showed a fairly linear relationship. The MHO score, when compared to the other two scores, had a more sigmoid shaped curve than linear suggesting that at the extremes, the MHO scores were clustered and not spread out like the M2 DASH and PEM scores. This implies that the MHO score is less sensitive at both extremes.

Conclusion

This paper does not aim to recommend any one measurement instrument over another, but to provide some basic information regarding questionnaires and an overall assessment of the practicalities and statistical analyses of commonly used region-specific patient-completed questionnaires used in the hand.

The choice of instrument to be used will depend on many factors including the project, population and setting, mode of administration, and time and financial constraints. This paper aims to help researchers identify the advantages and disadvantages of two commonly using hand questionnaires.

References

Atroshi, I., Gummesson, C., Johnsson, R., Sprinchorn, A. (1999). Symptoms, disability and quality of life in patients with carpal tunnel syndrome. *J. Hand Surg.* 24A: 398-404.

Baldry Currens, J. A. (2000). Evaluation of disability and handicap following injury. *Injury*. 31: 99-106.

Beaton, D. E., Katz, J. N., Fossel, A. H., Wright, J. G., Tarasuk, V., Bombardier, C. (2001). Measuring the whole or the parts? Validity, reliability, and responsiveness of the Disabilities of the Arm, Shoulder and Hand outcome measure in different regions of the upper extremity. *J. Hand Ther*. 14: 128-146.

Bowling, A. (1997). *Research Methods in Health*. Open University Press, Buckingham.

Bucher, C., Hume, K. I. (2002). Assessment following hand trauma: a review of some commonly employed methods. *Br. J. Hand Ther*. 7: 79-84.

Cano, S. J., Browne, J. P., Lamping, D. L., Roberts, A. H., McGrouther, D. A., Black, N. A. (2004). The Patient Outcomes of Surgery-Hand/Arm (POS-Hand/Arm): a new patient-based outcome measure. *J. Hand Surg*. 29: 477-485.

Chung, K. C., Pillsbury, M. S., Walters, M. R. (1998). Reliability and validity testing of the Michigan Hand Outcomes questionnaire. *J. Hand Surg*. 23 A: 575–587.

Cook, D., Guyatt, G., Juniper, E., Griffith, L., McIlroy, W., Willan, A., Jaeschke, R., Epstein, R. (1993). Interviewer versus self-administered questionnaires in developing health-related quality of life instrument for asthma. *J. Clin. Epidem*. 46: 529-534.

Dias, J. J., Bhowal, B., Wildin, C. J., Thompson, J. R. (2001). Assessing the outcome of disorders of the hand. Is the patient evaluation measure reliable, valid, responsive and without bias? *J. Bone Joint Surg*. 83B: 235-240.

Dias, J. J., Rajan, R. A., Thompson, J. R. (2008). Which questionnaire is best? The reliability, validity and ease of use of the patient evaluation measure, the disabilities of the arm, shoulder and hand and the Michigan hand outcome measure. *J. Hand Surg*. 33B: 9-17.

Drummond, A. S., Sampaio, R. F., Mancini, M. C., Kirkwood, R. N., Stamm, T. A. (2007). Linking the disabilities of arm, shoulder, and hand to the international classification of functioning, disability, and health. *J. Hand Ther*. 20: 336-344.

Forward, D. P., Sithole, J. S., Davis, T. R. (2007). The internal consistency and validity of the Patient Evaluation Measure for outcomes assessment in distal radius fractures. *J. Hand Surg*. 32B: 262-267.

Hobby, J. L., Watts, C., Elliot, D. (2005). Validity and responsiveness of the patient evaluation measure as an outcome measure for carpal tunnel syndrome. *J. Hand Surg.* 30B: 350-354.

Jupiter, J. B., Ring, D. (2002). Treatment of unreduced elbow dislocations with hinged external fixation. *J. Bone Joint Surg.* 84A: 1630-1635.

Khan, W., Jain, R., Dillon, B., Clarke, L., Fehily, M., Ravenscroft, M. (2008). The 'M2 DASH'-Manchester-modified Disabilities of Arm Shoulder and Hand score. *Hand* (NY). 3: 240-244.

Khan, W., Dillon, B., Agarwal, M., Fehily, M., Ravenscroft, M. (2009). The validity, reliability, responsiveness and bias of the Manchester-Modified Disabilities of Arm Shoulder and Hand score in hand injuries. *Hand* (NY) (in press).

MacDermid, J. C., Richards, R. S., Donner, A., Bellamy, N., Roth, J. H. (2000). Responsiveness of the short form-36, disability of the arm, shoulder, and hand questionnaire, patient-rated wrist evaluation, and physical impairment measurements in evaluating recovery after a distal radius fracture. *J. Hand Surg.* 25A: 330-340.

Macey, A. C., Burke, F. D., Abbott, K., Barton, N. J., Bradbury, E., Bradley, A., Bradley, M. J., Brady, O., Burt, A., Brown, P. (1995). Outcomes of hand surgery. British Society for Surgery of the Hand. *J. Hand Surg.* 20B: 841-855.

Massy-Westropp, N., Krishnan, J., Ahern, M. (2004). Comparing the AUSCAN Osteoarthritis Hand Index, Michigan Hand Outcomes Questionnaire, and Sequential Occupational Dexterity Assessment for patients with rheumatoid arthritis. *J. Rheumatol.* 31: 1996-2001.

McKee, M. D., Wild, L. M., Schemitsch, E. H. (2003). Midshaft malunion of the clavicle. *J. Bone Joint Surg.* 85A: 790-797.

Sharma, R., Dias, J. J. (2000). Validity and reliability of three generic outcome measures for hand disorders. *J. Hand Surg.* 25B: 593-600.

Streiner, D., Norman, G. (1994). *Health Measurement Scales.* Oxford: Oxford University Press.

Westphal, T. (2007). Reliability and responsiveness of the German version of the Disabilities of the Arm, Shoulder and Hand questionnaire (DASH). *Unfallchirurg.* 110: 548-552.

Wood-Dauphinee, S. (1999). Assessing quality of life in clinical research: from where have we come and where are we going? *J. Clin. Epidemiol.* 52: 355-363.

In: Carpal Tunnel Syndrome
Editor: Morton Ledford

ISBN: 978-1-63321-142-1
© 2014 Nova Science Publishers, Inc.

Chapter 6

The Manchester-Modified Dash Questionnaire

Wasim S. Khan, Ph.D.[1,*]
and Matthew A. Ravenscroft, FRCS[2]
[1]University College London Institute of Orthopaedics
and Musculoskeletal Sciences, Royal National
Orthopaedic Hospital, Stanmore, London, UK
[2]Department of Trauma and Orthopaedics,
Stockport NHS Foundation Trust, Stepping
Hill Hospital, Stockport, UK

Abstract

Injuries and disease commonly affect the upper limb and these can significantly affect the ability of an individual to perform activities of daily living.

The use of regional outcome measures or scoring systems is important as it allows comparison between these injuries and disease, and allows clinicians to assess progression and the effects of different treatment modalities. A patient-completed questionnaire is efficient in

---

* Corresponding author: Mr. Wasim S. Khan, Academic Clinical Fellow, University College London Institute of Orthopaedics and Musculoskeletal Science, Royal National Orthopaedic Hospital, Stanmore, London, HA7 4LP, UK. Telephone number: +44 (0) 7971 190720, Fax number: +44 (0) 20 8570 3864, E-mail address: wasimkhan@doctors.org.uk.

terms of time and resources, and allows the assessment of outcome without the need to attend an outpatient clinic.

It is important that the scoring system allows satisfactory regional outcome measurements specific for the upper limb. This is particularly important in injuries and disease that involve both upper and lower limbs.

The validity, reliability, responsiveness and bias are used for the assessment of various questionnaires. There are also many practical issues concerning the use of questionnaires including feasibility of use for the patient and the clinician.

The Disability of the Arm, Shoulder and Hand (DASH) questionnaire is a region-specific outcome measures commonly used for the upper limb, and is a patient-completed questionnaire. It is frequently used to assess self-reported patient outcome in orthopaedics, rheumatology and neurology. In this paper the DASH questionnaire is discussed along with its disadvantages that lead the authors to create the Manchester-Modified DASH.

With an increasing number of treatment modalities becoming available, and with the emphasis on evidence-based practice, there is an ever-increasing use of regional outcome measures used in the assessment of patients to identify the optimal treatment modality.

These questionnaires are useful as they do not provide limited information about one modality e.g. pain or function, but rather provide a single measure for multiple modalities. It also encompasses a range of symptoms including the physical, social and psychological.

It is important that hand surgeons and other disciplines involved with the care of patients with hand injury and disease have an understanding of the commonly used hand questionnaires.

The Disability of the Arm, Shoulder and Hand (DASH) questionnaire was developed for use in North America (Beaton et al., 2001) but translated versions have been validated in a number of languages including French and Japanese (Imaeda et al., 2005), Spanish (Hervás et al., 2006) and German (Westphal, 2007).

The Disability of the Arm, Shoulder and Hand (DASH) questionnaire (Hudak et al., 1996) is probably the most commonly used patient-completed regional outcome measure used for the hand (Khan et al., 2004; Khan and Fahmy, 2006). The main developmental objective was to develop a patient-reported regional outcome measure which considers the upper limb as a single functional unit allowing greater uniformity. The DASH questionnaire measures symptoms and functional status in patients with disorders of the upper limb. It was originally designed and validated as a measure of disability in patients with upper limb disorders.

The DASH questionnaire is used in orthopaedics, rheumatology and neurology to assess self-reported patient outcome (Jupiter and Ring, 2002; McKee et al., 2003).

Development of the DASH Questionnaire

During the development of the questionnaire, 13 scales and 821 items used in measuring the outcomes of various upper limb conditions were chosen after an extensive literature review. Staged item reduction was performed based on expert opinion to 177 items, based on content experts to 75 items, and following pilot testing to 30 items. This includes 21 physical function items, 6 symptom items and 3 social function items. The six domains assessed in the DASH questionnaire are daily activities, symptoms, social function, work function, sleep and confidence. There are also two optional modules, the high performance sports module and the work module.

The score out of 100 is calculated from the questionnaire after the patient answers 30 questions, evaluating symptoms and physical function, choosing one of five responses from a five-point Likert scale.

The final score is calculated using the formula below

DASH score= ((Average response per question answered) - 1) x 25

The DASH questionnaire allows for the omission of up to three questions. It is a time-consuming outcome measure and takes the patient 10 to 15 minutes to complete, and the clinician 5 minutes to calculate the final score.

Statistical Analyses

In 2001, Beaton et al. studied 200 patients with either, wrist and hand or shoulder problems to determine the validity, test-retest reliability and responsiveness of the DASH questionnaire. Correlations or t-tests between the DASH and the other measures were used to assess construct validity. Beaton et al. found the DASH questionnaire to correlate well with other measures including the Brigham questionnaire, the Shoulder Pain and Disability Index (SPADI) and other markers of pain and function (r > 0.69). Eighty-six patients completed a further questionnaire after three to five days and test-retest reliability was determined by intra-class correlation coefficient (ICC=0.96).

Responsiveness was determined using the standardised response means and correlations between change in DASH questionnaire score and change in scores of other measures, and showed that the responsiveness of the DASH was either comparable with or better than the joint-specific measures. The

DASH was shown to be responsive with changes found to correlate well with changes in the patient's condition. The standardised response mean of 0.74 for the DASH questionnaire was comparable to 0.76 for joint specific outcome measures e.g. the Brigham score.

The DASH questionnaire has a good correlation with the International Classification of Functioning, Disability and Health (Drummond et al., 2007). The DASH questionnaire has also been shown to have a good correlation with radiological and objective physical results (Wilcke et al., 2007). The DASH questionnaire showed convergent validity through a correlation with other joint specific instruments, such as the Brigham Carpal Tunnel Questionnaire (0.73) and the Shoulder Pain and Disability Index (0.72). It has shown validity and responsiveness in both proximal and distal disorders suggesting usefulness in all upper limb disorders (Beaton et al., 2001).

The DASH questionnaire showed a weaker correlation with severity of pain in the wrist joint (0.67) suggesting that it was less valid for use in patients with wrist injuries or disease.

The DASH questionnaire has been shown to be reliable with a Cronbach's alpha of 0.90-0.97 in a number of studies suggesting good internal consistency (Van de Ven-Stevens et al., 2009). The test–retest reliability was assessed in 86 patients who were asked to complete the questionnaire at baseline and then three to five days later. The Pearson correlation between the baseline and retest scores was 0.96 suggesting excellent reproducibility.

In other studies the DASH questionnaire showed an interclass correlation coefficient of 0.95 and 0.96 for a total population of 88 and 56 patients respectively, and a Pearson correlation coefficient of 0.98 for the total DASH scores of the initial assessment and the reassessment in 50 patients (Van de Ven-Stevens et al., 2009).

Disadvantages of the DASH Questionnaire

It was originally developed as a regional outcome measure specific for the upper limb but recent studies showed that patients with lower limb disability had DASH scores higher than normal control subjects (Dowrick et al., 2006; Khan et al., 2008).

This suggests that the questionnaire does not exclusively measure disability associated with disorders of the upper limb. This means that in studies looking at DASH scores where there were injuries to both upper and lower limbs, and in studies of polyarthropathies, the DASH scores need to be interpreted with caution.

A study investigating the construct validity of the DASH questionnaire was performed to determine whether the questionnaire measures disability solely attributed to the upper limb (Khan et al., 2008). One hundred and ninety two patients completed the DASH questionnaire, including 79 patients with upper limb injuries, 61 patients with lower limb injuries and 52 control subjects.

The DASH scores were calculated and comparisons of the scores between the three groups were made using the Kruskal-Wallis test. Pairwise comparisons between the groups were also made using the Mann-Whitney test. The mean DASH scores and standard deviations for the three groups were 54 (22) for the upper limb group, 16 (10) for the lower limb group, and 2 (3) for the control group, and the scores varied significantly between the three groups (Kruskal-Wallis: $p<0.001$).

The mean score for the upper limb group were higher than the lower limb group (Mann-Whitney: $p<0.001$), and the mean score for the lower limb group was higher than the control group (Mann-Whitney: $p<0.001$) (Figure 1).

Patients with lower limb pathologies who completed the DASH questionnaire scored significantly higher than the control suggesting that the questions are not specific for the upper limb.

This was because the DASH questionnaire includes questions that do not solely rely on the function of the upper limb e.g. 'ability to make a bed' or 'ability to manage transportation needs'.

These questions thus address both lower and upper limb disability. Other questions in the DASH questionnaire do not involve the use of the lower limb function e.g. 'ability to turn a key' or 'ability to open a jar'.

Statistical analyses of the original DASH questionnaire has also showed a high internal consistency (Dias et al., 2008) suggesting redundancy in questions.

The original DASH questionnaire also has other limitations. It is difficult to reproduce as it spans four pages, it is somewhat lengthy with 30 questions, the completion of the optional modules is variable, and importantly it is not specific for the upper limb. These issues prompted the authors to create a modified shorter version, the M^2 DASH that is more specific for the upper limb.

Manchester-Modified Disability of the Arm, Shoulder and Hand (M^2 DASH) questionnaire

Patient's Name/ Reference.. Date................................

Clinician's Name/ Reference..

INSTRUCTIONS FOR PATIENT: This questionnaire asks about your symptoms as well as you ability to perform certain activities. Please answer every question, based on your condition in the last week. If you did not have the opportunity to perform an activity in the past week, please make your best estimate on which response would be the most accurate. It doesn't matter which hand or arm you use to perform the activity; please answer based on you ability regardless of how you perform the task.

Please rate your ability to do the following activities in the last week.	No difficulty	Mild difficulty	Moderate difficulty	Severe difficulty	Unable
1. Open a tight or new jar	1	2	3	4	5
2. Write	1	2	3	4	5
3. Turn a key	1	2	3	4	5
4. Prepare a meal	1	2	3	4	5
5. Place an object on a shelf above your head	1	2	3	4	5
6. Wash or blow dry your hair	1	2	3	4	5
7. Wash your back	1	2	3	4	5
8. Put on a pullover sweater	1	2	3	4	5
9. Use a knife to cut food	1	2	3	4	5
10. Recreational activities which require little effort (eg cardplaying, knitting, etc)	1	2	3	4	5
11. Sexual activities	1	2	3	4	5
	Not at all	Slightly	Moderately	Quite a bit	Extremely
12. During the past week, to what extent has your arm, shoulder or hand problem interfered with your normal social activities with family, friends, neighbours or groups?	1	2	3	4	5
	Not limited at all	Slightly limited	Moderately limited	Very limited	Unable
13. During the past week, were you limited in your work or other regular daily activities as a result of your arm, shoulder or hand problem?	1	2	3	4	5
14. Tingling (pins and needles) in your arm, shoulder or hand	1	2	3	4	5
15. Weakness in your arm, shoulder or hand	1	2	3	4	5
16. Stiffness in your arm, shoulder or hand	1	2	3	4	5
	No difficulty	Mild difficulty	Moderate difficulty	Severe difficulty	So much difficulty I can't sleep
17. During the past week, how much difficulty have you had sleeping because of the pain in your arm, shoulder or hand?	1	2	3	4	5
	Strongly disagree	Disagree	Neither agree or disagree	Agree	Strongly agree
18. I feel less capable, less confident or less useful because of my arm, shoulder or hand problem	1	2	3	4	5

Thank you very much for completing all the questions in this questionnaire.

INSTRUCTIONS FOR CLINICIAN: The questionnaire can only be used if at least 16 out of the 18 questions have been answered. Using the formula below, you get a score out of 100.

$$\left(\left(\frac{\text{SUM OF TOTAL SCORE}}{\text{NUMBER OF QUESTIONS ANSWERED}}\right) \text{SUBTRACT 1}\right) \text{MULTIPLY BY 25} \quad = \quad \text{......................}$$

Reference: Khan, W. S., Jain, R., Dillon, B., Clarke, L., Fehily, M., Ravenskroft, M., (2008). *Hand*; 3(3):240-244.

Figure 1. M^2 DASH questionnaire in the one-page format including the instructions for patients and clinicians, and the equation for score calculation.

Manchester-Modified Disabilities of the Arm Shoulder and Hand Questionnaire

There are many outcome measures described in literature but not many are specific to the hand. The Disabilities of Arm, Shoulder and Hand (DASH) questionnaire was developed as a region specific outcome measure for the upper limb. A recent study however has shown that the DASH questionnaire is not specific for the upper limb and also measures disability in the lower limb (Khan et al., 2008).

A modified DASH score was created with fewer questions that can discriminate clearly between disabilities due to problems at the upper limb, and was more specific to the upper limb (Khan et al., 2008). The M^2 DASH questionnaire is not limited by lower limb pathologies and is more sensitive and specific for the upper limb. In isolated upper limb injuries the M^2 DASH questionnaire shows a good correlation with the original DASH questionnaire (Khan et al., 2008). This questionnaire could satisfactorily be used in patients with both upper and lower limb disability, and only measure the disability in the upper limb.

One hundred and ninety two patients completed the DASH questionnaire, including 79 patients with upper limb injuries, 61 patients with lower limb injuries and 52 control subjects.

The DASH scores were calculated and showed significant differences between the upper injury group, the lower injury group and the control group. The scores of the lower injury group were significantly higher than the control group suggesting that the DASH score measures disability attributed to the lower limb.

Using the frequency tables and bar charts for the scores for each group for each question, questions that the lower limb injury group scored highly on were identified and eliminated, resulting in the revised Manchester-Modified or M^2 DASH questionnaire containing questions specific to the upper limb (Table 1). The M^2 DASH questionnaire thus included questions 1-4, 6, 13-17, 21-23 and 26-30 from the original questionnaire and is shown in Figure 1. The revised questionnaire retains at least half the number of questions from each of the six domains described in the original DASH questionnaire.

It allows the omission of up to two questions and the score is calculated just like the original questionnaire by adding up the total scores from all answered questions, dividing it by the number of answered questions, subtracting 1 and multiplying by 25.

Table 1. The original DASH, QuickDASH and M² DASH questionnaires. The table shows the 30 questions that form the original DASH questionnaire

Please rate your ability to do the following activities in the last week.	No difficulty	Mild difficulty	Moderate difficulty	Severe difficulty	Unable
1. Open a tight or new jar	1	2	3	4	5
2. Write	1	2	3	4	5
3. Turn a key	1	2	3	4	5
4. Prepare a meal	1	2	3	4	5
5. Push open a heavy door	1	2	3	4	5
6. Place an object on a shelf above your head	1	2	3	4	5
7. Do heavy household chores (e.g. wash walls, wash floors)	1	2	3	4	5
8. Garden or do yard work	1	2	3	4	5
9. Make a bed	1	2	3	4	5
10. Carry a shopping bag or briefcase	1	2	3	4	5
11. Carry a heavy object (over 10 lbs)	1	2	3	4	5
12. Change a light bulb overhead	1	2	3	4	5
13. Wash or blow dry your hair	1	2	3	4	5
14. Wash your back	1	2	3	4	5
15. Put on a pullover sweater	1	2	3	4	5
16. Use a knife to cut food	1	2	3	4	5
17. Recreational activities which require little effort (e.g. cardplaying, knitting, etc.)	1	2	3	4	5
18. Recreational activities in which you take some force or impact through your arm, shoulder or hand (e.g. golf, hammering, tennis, etc.)	1	2	3	4	5

Please rate your ability to do the following activities in the last week.	No difficulty	Mild difficulty	Moderate difficulty	Severe difficulty	Unable
19. Recreational activities in which you move your arm freely (e.g. playing frisbee, badminton, etc.)	1	2	3	4	5
20. Manage transportation needs (getting from one place to another)	1	2	3	4	5
21. Sexual activities	1	2	3	4	5
	Not at all	Slightly	Moderately	Quite a bit	Extremely
22. During the past week, to what extent has your arm, shoulder or hand problem interfered with your normal social activities with family, friends, neighbours or groups?	1	2	3	4	5
	Not limited at all	Slightly limited	Moderately limited	Very limited	Unable
23. During the past week, were you limited in your work or other regular daily activities as a result of your arm, shoulder or hand problem?	1	2	3	4	5
Please rate the severity of the following symptoms in the last week	None	Mild	Moderate	Severe	Extreme
24. Arm, shoulder or hand pain	1	2	3	4	5
25. Arm, shoulder or hand pain when you performed any specific activity	1	2	3	4	5
26. Tingling (pins and needles) in your arm, shoulder or hand	1	2	3	4	5
27. Weakness in your arm, shoulder or hand	1	2	3	4	5
28. Stiffness in your arm, shoulder or hand	1	2	3	4	5

Table 1. (Continued)

Please rate your ability to do the following activities in the last week.	No difficulty	Mild difficulty	Moderate difficulty	Severe difficulty	Unable
	No difficulty	Mild difficulty	Moderate difficulty	Severe difficulty	So much difficulty I can't sleep
29. During the past week, how much difficulty have you had sleeping because of the pain in your arm, shoulder or hand?	1	2	3	4	5
	Strongly disagree	Disagree	Neither agree or disagree	Agree	Strongly agree
30. I feel less capable, less confident or less useful because of my arm, shoulder or hand problem	1	2	3	4	5

The QuickDASH questions are highlighted in italics and the M^2 DASH questions are highlighted in bold. The score is calculated by adding up the total scores for each answered question, dividing it by the number of answered questions, subtracting 1 and multiplying by 25. This applies to all three questionnaires and gives a score out of 100 (Khan et al., 2008).

Comparison of the M^2 DASH scores between the three groups was also made using the Kruskal-Wallis test, followed by pair-wise comparisons between the groups using the Mann-Whitney test. The mean M^2 DASH scores and standard deviations for the three groups were 51 (23) for the upper limb group, 9 (9) for the lower limb group, and 2 (2) for the control group. The M^2 DASH scores varied significantly between the three groups (Kruskal-Wallis: $p<0.001$). Pair-wise comparisons between the upper and lower limb groups (Mann-Whitney: $p<0.001$), and between the upper limb and control groups (Mann-Whitney: $p<0.001$) showed statistically significant differences.

Importantly, no significant difference was seen between the lower limb group and the control group (Mann-Whitney: $p>0.05$) when using the M^2 DASH scores unlike the DASH scores. Using chi-square tests, only question 10 ($p>0.05$) and question 20 ($p>0.05$) showed no evidence of a difference between the upper limb and lower limb group, suggesting that they were not specific for the upper limb group.

These two questions were not in the M^2 DASH questionnaire. The M^2 DASH questionnaire score was then calculated for the group of patients with upper limb injury and a correlation study performed with the original DASH questionnaire score to assess the validity of the modified questionnaire.

This showed a high correlation (Spearman's correlation coefficient, r=0.98, p<0.001) confirming that the ranking of the upper limb patients is similar in the two questionnaires.

The authors of the study developed the M^2 DASH after excluding questions that were not specific to the upper limb. The purpose of developing the M^2 DASH questionnaire was to devise a questionnaire that is more specific for upper limb injuries and disease.

The M^2 DASH questionnaire was devised by excluding twelve questions from the DASH questionnaire that were not specific for the upper limb including 'ability to carry a shopping bag or briefcase' and 'ability to manage transportation needs'. In the modified questionnaire, at least half the questions from the original questionnaire's six domains remain.

The questionnaire allows for the omission of up to two questions and the score is adjusted to accommodate for this. The study describing the M^2 DASH questionnaire showed a significant correlation between the scores obtained using the original and revised questionnaires in the group with upper limb injury also suggesting that the revised questionnaire is valid.

The M^2 DASH questionnaire has construct validity as the questionnaire retains at least half of the questions from each of the six domains of the original DASH questionnaire (Khan et al., 2008).

The M^2 DASH questionnaire includes some questions that do not form part of the routine objective assessments of the hand, suggesting good content or face validity.

As the only previous assessment of the validity of the M^2 DASH question-naire was by comparison with the original DASH questionnaire from which the M^2 DASH scores had been extrapolated, a more thorough investigation was needed.

It is important to determine the validity, reliability, responsiveness and bias of the newly created M2 DASH questionnaire. The validity establishes whether the outcome measure actually measures what it has been designed to.

An outcome tool is reliable if the same score is obtained at different time points after the clinical condition has stabilised. The responsiveness is the ability to detect clinically important changes at different intervals. Bias can occur when variables assumed to be independent, such as age and gender, affect scores.

The Patient Evaluation Measure (PEM) questionnaire was developed in the UK in 1995 (Macey et al., 1995), and the Michigan Hand Outcome (MHO) questionnaire was developed in the US in 1998 (Chung et al., 1998).

Both questionnaires are patient-completed region-specific outcome measures commonly used for hand injuries. In a more recent study we assessed the validity, reliability, responsiveness and bias of the M^2 DASH questionnaire for hand injuries using completed M^2 DASH, PEM and MHO questionnaires (Khan et al., in press).

Fifty nine patients with hand injuries who completed the M^2 DASH and MHO questionnaires at their first clinic visit, on discharge following their last visit, and at six months following discharge were studied. Patients were also asked to complete the M^2 DASH 12 months following discharge. Nine patients were lost to follow-up, six had a further injury or a recurrence of the previous injury, and four had inadequately completed questionnaires.

Questionnaires from the remaining 40 patients with injuries to the hand were used to assess the validity, reliability, responsiveness and bias of the M^2 DASH questionnaire.

The M^2 DASH, PEM and MHO scores were then calculated.

The validity of the M^2 DASH was assessed by determining how well the questionnaire score correlated with the PME and MHO scores. Using histograms it was determined that the scores were normally distributed, and Pearson correlations were used to compare the scores. Criterion validity testing showed strong correlations between the M^2 DASH scores and the PME and MHO scores suggesting that the M^2 DASH score measures what it is designed to and confirmed that the questionnaire is valid for injuries to the hand. The M^2 DASH scores showed highly significant positive correlations with the PEM and MHO scores at all three time points ($p<0.001$).

The magnitude of the correlation coefficient was slightly lower with the MHO scores than the PEM scores, and at six months following discharge than earlier.

The reliability was determined by performing test-retest analyses on the M^2 DASH scores at six and 12 months following discharge. Six months following discharge, as the patients had not sustained any further injury or sought further medical advice for the original injury, it was assumed that their condition had stabilised. There was a statistically significant correlation between the M^2 DASH scores six months and 12 months following discharge ($r=0.73$, $p<0.001$) suggesting good test-retest reproducibility and reliability.

Responsiveness was determined by correlating the changes in the M^2 DASH score with changes in the PEM and MHO scores.

This was done by calculating the effect size and the standardised response mean. The effect sizes were calculated by dividing the mean of change in the scores during the period from initial presentation to discharge, and from discharge to six months following discharge, by the standard deviation of the baseline score. The standardised response mean was calculated by dividing the mean of change in the scores between initial presentation and six months following discharge by the standard deviation of the change in score. The effect sizes for the M^2 DASH scores were 1.45 and 1.07 for the time periods between presentation and discharge, and between discharge and six months following discharge respectively. These values were greater than 0.8 suggesting that they were valuable. The effect sizes for the two periods were greater than those for the PME scores (1.26 and 0.96) and MHO scores (1.23 and 0.60). The effect size for the MHO scores between discharge and six months following discharge was less than 0.80 suggesting that they were not valuable. The standardised response means for the M^2 DASH, PME and MHO scores were 2.21, 1.80 and 1.50 respectively, suggesting that the M^2 DASH is a highly responsive scale. This study established that the M^2 DASH questionnaire is responsive to change compared with the PME and MHO questionnaires from initial presentation following injury through discharge from the fracture clinic and to 6 months following discharge.

The bias was investigated by performing correlation studies for assumed independent variables including age, gender, hand dominance, the side injured. There was no association between the M^2 DASH scores at presentation and 12 months following discharge, and gender, dominance and injury to dominant side confirming no bias. There was evidence of a weak association between age and the M^2 DASH score at presentation but the correlation coefficient was not large (r=0.37, p=0.02). The positive correlation implies that older patients have higher DASH scores when they present with hand injuries. There are two possible explanations for this. Either older patients sustain more severe hand injuries or sustain injuries of similar severity but suffer a greater disability as a result of the injury. Although the latter explanation is more likely, further work is needed to explore this in more detail. There was no correlation at 12 months following discharge (r=-0.09, p=0.57).

Initial studies suggest that the M^2 DASH questionnaire is a robust region specific outcome measure. It is a valid and responsive questionnaire with test-retest reliability proven for hand injuries. Gender, handedness and side injured did not cause bias in the responses. There is a need for further studies looking beyond hand injuries before a more complete picture on the validity of the M^2 DASH for all upper limb pathologies could be drawn.

The M^2 DASH is an upper limb outcome assessment tool that is not pathology or region specific within the upper limb. It has a simple one-page layout and is easy to understand and complete for the patient.

For the researcher, it is easy to enter into a database, and to calculate and analyse the score.

Conclusion

This chapter does not recommend any one measurement instrument over another, but to provide some basic information regarding the DASH questionnaires, and an overall assessment of the practicalities and statistical analyses of this region-specific patient-completed questionnaire commonly used in the assessment of the upper limb.

References

Atroshi, I., Gummesson, C., Johnsson, R., Sprinchorn, A. (1999). Symptoms, disability and quality of life in patients with carpal tunnel syndrome. *J. Hand Surg.* 24A: 398-404.

Baldry Currens, J. A. (2000). Evaluation of disability and handicap following injury. *Injury.* 31: 99-106.

Beaton, D. E., Katz, J. N., Fossel, A. H., Wright, J. G., Tarasuk, V., Bombardier, C. (2001). Measuring the whole or the parts? Validity, reliability, and responsiveness of the Disabilities of the Arm, Shoulder and Hand outcome measure in different regions of the upper extremity. *J. Hand Ther.* 14: 128-146.

Bowling, A. (1997). *Research Methods in Health.* Open University Press, Buckingham.

Bucher, C., Hume, K. I. (2002). Assessment following hand trauma: a review of some commonly employed methods. *Br. J. Hand Ther.* 7: 79-84.

Dias, J. J., Rajan, R. A., Thompson, J. R. (2008). Which questionnaire is best? The reliability, validity and ease of use of the patient evaluation measure, the disabilities of the arm, shoulder and hand and the Michigan hand outcome measure. *J. Hand Surg.* 33B: 9-17.

Dowrick, A. S., Gabbe, B. J., Williamson, O. D., Cameron, P. A. (2006). Does the disabilities of the arm, shoulder and hand (DASH) scoring system only measure disability due to injuries to the upper limb? *J. Bone Joint Surg.* 88B: 524-527.

Drummond, A. S., Sampaio, R. F., Mancini, M. C., Kirkwood, R. N., Stamm, T. A. (2007). Linking the disabilities of arm, shoulder, and hand to the international classification of functioning, disability, and health. *J. Hand Ther.* 20: 336-344.

Hervás, M. T., Navarro Collado, M. J., Peiró, S., Rodrigo Pérez, J. L., López Matéu, P., Martínez Tello, I. (2006). Spanish version of the DASH questionnaire. Cross-cultural adaptation, reliability, validity and responsiveness. *Med. Clin.* (Barc.). 127: 441-447.

Imaeda, T., Toh, S., Nakao, Y., Nishida, J., Hirata, H., Ijichi, M., Kohri, C., Nagano, A.; for the Impairment Evaluation Committee, Japanese Society for Surgery of the Hand (2005). Validation of the Japanese Society for Surgery of the Hand version of the Disability of the Arm, Shoulder, and Hand questionnaire. *J. Orthop. Sci.* 10: 353-359.

Jupiter, J. B., Ring, D. (2002). Treatment of unreduced elbow dislocations with hinged external fixation. *J. Bone Joint Surg.* 84A: 1630-1635.

Khan, W. S., Agarwal, M., Muir, L. (2004). Management of intra-articular fractures of the proximal interphalangeal joint with internal fixation and bone grafting. *Arch. Orthop. Trauma Surg.* 124: 654-658.

Khan, W. S., Fahmy, N. R. M. (2006). The S-Quattro in the management of sports injuries of the hand. *Injury.* 37: 860-868.

Khan, W., Jain, R., Dillon, B., Clarke, L., Fehily, M., Ravenscroft, M. (2008). The 'M2 DASH'-Manchester-modified Disabilities of Arm Shoulder and Hand score. *Hand* (NY). 3: 240-244.

Khan, W., Dillon, B., Agarwal, M., Fehily, M., Ravenscroft, M. (2009). The validity, reliability, responsiveness and bias of the Manchester-Modified Disabilities of Arm Shoulder and Hand score in hand injuries. *Hand* (NY) (in press).

MacDermid, J. C., Richards, R. S., Donner, A., Bellamy, N., Roth, J. H. (2000). Responsiveness of the short form-36, disability of the arm, shoulder, and hand questionnaire, patient-rated wrist evaluation, and physical impairment measurements in evaluating recovery after a distal radius fracture. *J. Hand Surg.* 25A: 330-340.

Macey, A. C., Burke, F. D., Abbott, K., Barton, N. J., Bradbury, E., Bradley, A., Bradley, M. J., Brady, O., Burt, A., Brown, P. (1995). Outcomes of hand surgery. British Society for Surgery of the Hand. *J. Hand Surg.* 20B: 841-855.

McKee, M. D., Wild, L. M., Schemitsch, E. H. (2003). Midshaft malunion of the clavicle. *J. Bone Joint Surg.* 85A: 790-797.

Sharma, R., Dias, J. J. (2000). Validity and reliability of three generic outcome measures for hand disorders. *J. Hand Surg.* 25B: 593-600.

Streiner, D., Norman, G. (1994). *Health Measurement Scales.* Oxford: Oxford University Press.

Westphal, T. (2007). Reliability and responsiveness of the German version of the Disabilities of the Arm, Shoulder and Hand questionnaire (DASH). *Unfallchirurg.* 110: 548-552.

Wilcke, M. K., Abbaszadegan, H., Adolphson, P. Y. (2007). Patient-perceived outcome after displaced distal radius fractures: a comparison between radiological parameters, objective physical variables, and the DASH score. *J. Hand Ther.* 20: 290-299.

In: Carpal Tunnel Syndrome
Editor: Morton Ledford

ISBN: 978-1-63321-142-1
© 2014 Nova Science Publishers, Inc.

Chapter 7

Carpal Tunnel Syndrome: Epidemiology and Risk Factors

Sergio Gennaro, M.D., Pietro Fiaschi, M.D. *
and Paolo Merciadri, M.D.

Department of Neurosurgery, San Martino -
IST University Hospital (IRCCS), Genoa, Italy

Abstract

Carpal tunnel syndrome (CTS) is the most frequent mononeuropathy seen in the general population. Defined as median nerve compression at the level of the wrist, CTS causes numbness and tingling in the hand and fingers. The first introduction of the term "carpal tunnel syndrome" is attributed to Brain in 1947 and the popularization of its diagnosis and treatment to Phalen in 1950. Since then, there has been continued debate over the optimal management of this disease. CTS is the most expensive upper-extremity musculoskeletal disorder at an estimated cost of medical care in the US exceeding $2 billion annually, primarily due to surgical releases. The extra-medical costs are substantially greater. In fact, during 2006 in the US, surgeons performed 580,000 outpatient carpal tunnel releases [6] and the median lost worktime from work-related CTS is 27

* Corresponding author: Pietro Fiaschi, M.D. Department of Neurosurgery, San Martino - IST University Hospital (IRCCS), Largo Rosanna Benzi 10, 16132 Genoa, Italy. Phone + 39. 3402767717, E-mail: pietro.fiaschi@alice.it.

days, which is longer than any other work-related disorder except fractures. Although CTS is a strong driver of workers compensation costs, lost wages, lost productivity, and disability, there is still an incomplete understanding of its frequency and causes in working populations. Prevalent CTS in general populations range from 1–5% and among manufacturing and meat-packing workers has ranged from 5–21%.

Incidence rates from many studies on workers of CTS ranged from 1–15 per 1000 person-years and varied by industrial and occupational. In the general population, the emphasis on possibly risk factors is focused on demographic characteristics (female gender, older age) and on comorbid conditions (higher BMI, rheumatoid arthritis, diabetes mellitus and thyroid disease. Associations between CTS and other risk factors, such as gout, smoking status are uncertain as well as personal and workplace psychosocial possible involvement. However, general population studies do not take workplace exposures into account. The prevalence of CTS in working populations is generally higher than in the general population. Occupation-related CTS represents one of the major health problems among workers in various occupations throughout the world including Sweden, Italy, France, Japan, Taiwan. Recognized occupational risk factors are identify manual loadings with a significantly higher risk or association with CTS, comprise the use of handheld vibrating machinery, forceful gripping of objects with hands, repetitive and frequent manual tasks and forced postures of the wrist (flexion/extension). These loadings are usually combined during occupational work.

Epidemiology

Carpal tunnel syndrome (CTS) is the most frequent mononeuropathy seen in the general population. The first introduction of the term "carpal tunnel syndrome" is attributed to Brain in 1947 and the popularization of its diagnosis and treatment to Phalen in 1950 [8, 25-27].

Before introducing statistical and epidemiologic data it is necessary to point out a concern regarding the selection of an appropriate inclusive criteria. Case definitions with the greatest possible sensitivity and specificity are preferred for epidemiologic research as well as for clinical applications. At present, there is not a perfect "Carpal tunnel Syndrome" gold standard, but the combination of a positive electrodiagnostic study and characteristic symptoms appears to have the best predictive value as a case definition of carpal tunnel syndrome.

In fact, case definitions using combinations of symptom characteristics and physical examination findings alone are likely to result in more misclassification of disease status.

On the other hand, the electrodiagnostic study alone, despite it is an "objective" test and presumably measures the underlying pathophysiologic process of the condition, provides several problems. Firstly, intraexaminer and interexaminer difference in reliability of measures of median nerve latency and velocity is high. In addition, carpal tunnel syndrome is, by definition, a clinical syndrome with a characteristic symptom complex and, in severe cases, clear physical examination findings. Case definitions based only on the electrodiagnostic study ignore these additional data that are likely to improve the accuracy of classification [31].

However, because the methods for case confirmation based on clinical and electrophysiologic criteria can be overly restrictive, the real incidence of carpal tunnel syndrome in many studies has been probably underestimated. Such cases could make up 5 to 10% of the total, depending on the sensitivity of the electrophysiologic tests used [19].

Incidence

In a Italian 8-year long study on general population, the mean annual standardized incidence of CTS diagnosed on the basis of clinical symptoms and delay in distal conduction velocity of the median nerve was 0,27 cases per 100 person-years. The sex-specific incidences were 0,13% for men and 0,5% for women. The mean annual incidence for men increased moderately but significantly during the study period, whereas that for women remained constant. The age-specific incidence for women increased gradually with age, reaching a peak between 50 and 59 years, after which it declined. In men instead, there was a bimodal distribution with peaks between 50 and 59 years and between 70 and 79 years [19].

In Sweden, the annual incidence of clinically diagnosed carpal tunnel syndrome was 0,43% in women and 0,18% in men, with a peak among women aged 45 to 54 years [3].

The annual age standardized rates of new presentations in primary care in United Kingdom, carpal tunnel syndrome represented the 0,08% for men and the 0,19% for women; the operative treatment was undertaken one third of new presentations of CTS [6, 17].

In France, hospital admissions for CTS surgery were identified in patients aged 20 years and older, giving an overall incidence of 2.7/1000 per year (females 3.6/1000, males 1.7/1000) [39].

A meta-analysis evaluated the pooled incidence in US working populations of carpal tunnel syndrome as 2.94% per year.

A retrospective, nationwide cohort study performed in Korea from 2005 to 2007 defined the incidence of total clinically diagnosed CTS and electrophysiologically diagnosed CTS in patients over 20 years of age was 4.96 and 0.98 per 1,000 person-years, respectively. The incidence of surgically treated CTS was 0.29 per 1,000 person-years. The female to male incidence ratio of diagnosed carpal tunnel syndrome was 2.6 and that of surgically treated CTS was 5.8. Women aged 50 to 59 years had the highest incidence of carpal tunnel syndrome, whereas men showed the highest at 60 to 69 years. Compared with Western studies, Korean population showed a similar incidence of CTS but a lower incidence of surgery. Korean women with CTS are more likely to be treated surgically than men [32].

Prevalence

Studies performed in Sweden estimated the prevalence of symptoms compatible with carpal tunnel syndrome in 14,4% of general population, and 2.7% the prevalence of clinically and electrophysiologically confirmed carpal tunnel syndrome [3].

Another study on Swedish general population individuated there is a 0.7% prevalence of undiagnosed CTS with a severity similar to that of patients undergoing surgery [4].

A scandinavian meta-analysis established the pooled prevalence of carpal tunnel syndrome is 7.09%.

In US, B Prevalent CTS in general populations range from 1–5% and among manufacturing and meat-packing workers has ranged from 5–21% [12].

Based on interviews distributed in 1988 in US, self-reported carpal tunnel syndrome involves 1,5% of adults. The prevalence among Whites was 1,8 times higher than non- Whites, and women had 1,6 times higher prevalence than men [37].

Other Features

CTS is a bilateral affection in 55-65% of cases [6]. Recurrence of carpal tunnel syndrome following surgery is not rare. The reported frequency of re-operation varies from 0.3 to 12% [30].

A seasonal distribution of CTS, which demonstrates a significant association with winter months, maybe due to the influence of cold temperatures on neuropathies [34].

Costs

Carpal tunnel syndrome (CTS) is a common cause of upper limb complaints with social implications caused by lost days of work, change of occupation, and high health care costs [37]. CTS is the most expensive upper-extremity musculoskeletal disorder at an estimated cost of medical care in the US exceeding $2 billion annually, primarily due to surgical releases. The extra-medical costs are substantially greater. In fact, CTS patients surgically treated in the United States number between 400,000 and 500,000 per year [14, 21, 33] and the median lost worktime from work-related CTS is 27 days, which is longer than any other work-related disorder except fractures. Although CTS is a strong driver of workers' compensation costs, lost wages, lost productivity, and disability, there is still an incomplete understanding of its frequency and causes in working populations. In 2007, the income loss per CTS patient over a period of 6 years was estimated at $45,000-89,000 in US [25, 26]. Prevalent CTS in general populations range from 1–5% and among manufacturing and meat-packing workers has ranged from 5–21%. Incidence rates from many studies on workers of CTS ranged from 1–15 per 1000 person-years and varied by industrial and occupational [12]. The prevalence of CTS in working populations is generally higher than in the general population. Occupation-related CTS represents one of the major health problems among workers in various occupations throughout the world including Sweden [4], Italy [5], France [18], Japan [20], Taiwan [10].

Recognized occupational risk factors are identify manual loadings with a significantly higher risk or association with CTS, comprise the use of handheld vibrating machinery, forceful gripping of objects with hands, repetitive and frequent manual tasks and forced postures of the wrist (flexion/extension). These loadings are usually combined during occupational work [36, 44].

Risk Factors

Multiple risk factors contribute to the occurrence of CTS. Indeed the incidence may be increased by biological, medical and work conditions.

Biological factors include increasing age, female sex [2, 16] and anatomical characteristics of the hand and the wrist [7]; medical conditions associated with CTS include obesity, inflammatory arthritis, diabetes mellitus, hypo-thyroidism, hemodialysis and leprosy [2, 7, 15, 16, 22, 35, 42]; work-related factors include prolonged or repeated forceful exertions, prolonged or repeated flexion or extensions of the wrist, use of vibratory tools and cold exposure [9, 22, 23, 28, 41]. See Table 1.

Which are the prevailing conditions? In most cases CTS seems to be a constitutional condition on which occupational activities play a detrimental additional role. The American Academy of Orthopaedic Surgeons also quantified a two-fold higher importance for biological factors [11].

Biological factors: in general population, female sex and increasing age are associated with CTS. During pregnancy CTS has been observed with a prevalence of 62% [1, 22].

Boz et al. found a correlation between wrist index (calculated by dividing depth by width), hand index (hand width (mm) × 100/hand length (mm)) and digit index (digit 3 length (mm) × 100/hand length (mm)) and CTS; in depth they obtained higher mean wrist indices in CTS patients when compared to control subjects and, in females, they found low hand indices and short digits to be significant risk factors for CTS [7].

Table 1. CTS risk factors

Biologic Factors	Medical factors	Work-related factors
Advanced age Female sex Pregnancy Hand/wrist anatomy	High BMI Inflammatory tenosynovitis Diabetes mellitus Hypothyroidism Hemodialysis Oral corticosteroids therapy Estrogen replacement therapy Acromegaly Gout / smoking status (uncertain) Leprosy	Forceful exertions Prolonged or repetitive flexion/extension of the wrist Vibratory tools Cold exposure Computer mouse usage (uncertain)

That is probably because while using the hand with these anatomic conditions, a higher pressure in the intracarpal area is exerted.

Medical factors: these are the commonly examined factors in general population.

Higher body mass index (BMI) score is a definite risk factor for CTS in both genders. Some researchers suggest that the mechanism is probably correlated to the increased fatty tissue and/or an increased hydrostatic pressure within the carpal canal [7, 16, 42].

Inflammatory tenosynovitis [2, 22, 35] and presumably any form of inflammation of wrist, joints or tendon sheaths can cause compression of the median nerve in the carpal tunnel. Inflammatory arthritis was associated with a nearly three-fold increase in risk of carpal tunnel surgery [35].

Diabetes mellitus is a known cause of CTS (40% increase in risk). The main mechanism is probably related to the diabetic vascular changes and tendinopathies, even if diabetic peripheral neuropathy can't be fully excluded with certainty [2, 22, 35].

Hypothyroidism was associated with a 70% increase in risk of CTS because of the myxedematous deposition and thickened synovial fluid in the carpal tunnel. Consumption of thyroid replacement medication was not found to increase the risk of CTS [2, 22, 35].

Hemodialysis is an important risk factor for CTS, associated with a nine-fold increase in risk probably due to median nerve entrapment caused by β_2-microglobulin amyloid deposition in the carpal tunnel [35].

The use of oral corticosteroids was associated with a 60% increased risk of CTS. This has been explained by three different mechanisms: their mineralocorticoid effect with expansion of fluid volume and generalized edema, possibly related hyperglycemia causing glycosylation of tissue end products, and the possible association with lipomatosis [35].

Increased risk of CTS has also been associated with estrogen replacement therapy (80% increase) [35] and with acromegaly [22], in which the median nerve is found to be swollen because of the excess of the growth hormone.

Gout and smoking status are two factors not clearly related to CTS; further investigation is needed [24, 29, 43].

In the rare subjects affected by leprosy, type I (reversal) reactions can lead to nerve swelling. If this happens within the carpal tunnel, external entrapment compression can be added to the internal pressure elevation generated by intraneural swelling, causing rapidly worsening, often bilateral, signs and symptoms of CTS [15]. Work-related factors: the prevalence of CTS in working populations is generally higher than in the general population.

Occupation-related CTS represents one of the major health problems among workers in various occupations throughout the world including Sweden [4], Italy [5], France [18], Japan [20], Taiwan [10].

Several authors studied carpal tunnel pressure (CTP), assuming that a persistent elevation in CTP can cause or aggravate CTS.

Moreover, CTP values were demonstrated to be higher for CTS patients than for healthy subjects [41].

Force results as the primary work-related risk factor: according to experimental studies the risk for CTS increases proportionally to the amount of time spent in activities associated with high force requirements of the hand. Particularly, CTP seems to be very sensitive to loading of the long flexors of the 1st, 2nd and 3rd digit [9, 41].

Additionally, external forces above the carpal tunnel area can lead to a considerably high CTP values, so that tool size and shape may be crucial factors in developing CTS [41].

Prolonged or repeated flexion and extension of the wrist has been consistently associated with a higher risk of CTS [23, 41]. Some authors associated a higher risk with wrist flexion or extension for at least half of the working day [22], others calculated a two-fold increase after one year in a job involving "repetitive wrist movement" or a six-fold increase in workers bending or twisting the hand or wrist "many times per hour" [23]. An elevated CTP was reported after flexion-extension exercise with a rate of 30 cycles per minute for 1 minute [41].

Exposure to hand-arm vibration is a clear risk factor for CTS, in fact in the United Kingdom this is the only situation in which CTS is considered an occupational disease. A more than doubling of risk was associated with a relatively prolonged and intense exposure [23].

CTS has also been consistently associated with cold exposure together with high repetitive wrist movements (14.39-fold risk compared with controls) [28]. The contribution of the single factors and the principal mechanism of cold exposure in the development of CTS remain unknown.

The association of CTS and the use of computer keyboard and mouse has also been studied: while the keyboard usage has not been clearly associated with an increased risk [22, 23, 38], an association was found with right-handed mouse usage [23].

The simultaneous presence of multiple risk factors, for example higher BMI and high physical job demands, increase the risk beyond what it would be if only one of the different factors was present. Global risk, that is, can't be calculated by simple sum of every single risk factor [9].

CTS in children must be mentioned as a rare occurrence often with an unusual presentation. It is more commonly associated with mucopolysaccharidosis and mucolipidosis. Other rare risk factors include diabetes mellitus, obesity, malformations of the hand, hemangiomatosis, trauma, osteoid osteomas and bleeding into the wrist (as in hemophilia). Familial carpal tunnel syndrome has also been reported in a few children probably as a consequence of an inheritable disorder of connective tissue mediated by an autosomal dominant gene [13, 40].

References

[1]   Ablove, R. H., Ablove, T. S. Prevalence of carpal tunnel syndrome in pregnant women. *WMJ* (2009) 108: 194-196.

[2]   Atcheson, S. G., Ward, J. R., Lowe, W. Concurrent medical disease in work-related carpal tunnel syndrome. *Arch. Intern. Med.* (1998) 158: 1506-1512.

[3]   Atroshi, I., Englund, M., Turkiewicz, A., Tagil, M., Petersson, I. F. Incidence of physician-diagnosed carpal tunnel syndrome in the general population. *Arch. Intern. Med.* (2011) 171: 943-944.

[4]   Atroshi, I., Gummesson, C., Johnsson, R., Ornstein, E., Ranstam, J., Rosen, I. Prevalence of carpal tunnel syndrome in a general population. *JAMA* (1999) 282: 153-158.

[5]   Baldasseroni, A., Tartaglia, R., Carnevale, F. [The risk of the carpal tunnel syndrome in some work activities]. *Med. Lav.* (1995) 86: 341-351.

[6]   Bland, J. D., Rudolfer, S. M. Clinical surveillance of carpal tunnel syndrome in two areas of the United Kingdom, 1991-2001. *J. Neurol. Neurosurg. Psychiatry* (2003) 74: 1674-1679.

[7]   Boz, C., Ozmenoglu, M., Altunayoglu, V., Velioglu, S., Alioglu, Z. Individual risk factors for carpal tunnel syndrome: an evaluation of body mass index, wrist index and hand anthropometric measurements. *Clin. Neurol. Neurosurg.* (2004) 106: 294-299.

[8]   Brain, W. R., Wright, A. D., Wilkinson, M. Spontaneous compression of both median nerves in the carpal tunnel; six cases treated surgically. *Lancet* (1947) 1: 277-282.

[9]   Burt, S., Deddens, J. A., Crombie, K., Jin, Y., Wurzelbacher, S., Ramsey, J. A prospective study of carpal tunnel syndrome: workplace and individual risk factors. *Occup. Environ. Med.* (2013) 70: 568-574.

[10] Chiang, H. C., Ko, Y. C., Chen, S. S., Yu, H. S., Wu, T. N., Chang, P. Y. Prevalence of shoulder and upper-limb disorders among workers in the fish-processing industry. *Scand. J. Work Environ. Health* (1993) 19: 126-131.

[11] Conolly, W. B., McKessar, J. H. Carpal tunnel syndrome-can it be a work related condition? *Aust. Fam. Physician* (2009) 38: 684-686.

[12] Dale, A. M., Harris-Adamson, C., Rempel, D., Gerr, F., Hegmann, K., Silverstein, B., Burt, S., Garg, A., Kapellusch, J., Merlino, L., Thiese, M. S., Eisen, E. A., Evanoff, B. Prevalence and incidence of carpal tunnel syndrome in US working populations: pooled analysis of six prospective studies. *Scand. J. Work Environ. Health* (2013) 39: 495-505.

[13] Davis, L., Vedanarayanan, V. V. Carpal tunnel syndrome in children. *Pediatr. Neurol.* (2014) 50: 57-59.

[14] Foley, M., Silverstein, B., Polissar, N. The economic burden of carpal tunnel syndrome: long-term earnings of CTS claimants in Washington State. *Am. J. Ind. Med.* (2007) 50: 155-172.

[15] Gennaro, S., Secci, F., Fiaschi, P., Merciadri, P. Supraorbital nerve entrapment neuropathy in Hansen's disease. *Neurol. Sci.* (2013) 34: 2243-2244.

[16] Komurcu, H. F., Kilic, S., Anlar, O. Relationship of Age, Body Mass Index, Wrist and Waist Circumferences to Carpal Tunnel Syndrome Severity. *Neurol. Med. Chir.* (Tokyo) (2013).

[17] Latinovic, R., Gulliford, M. C., Hughes, R. A. Incidence of common compressive neuropathies in primary care. *J. Neurol. Neurosurg. Psychiatry* (2006) 77: 263-265.

[18] Leclerc, A., Franchi, P., Cristofari, M. F., Delemotte, B., Mereau, P., Teyssier-Cotte, C., Touranchet, A. Carpal tunnel syndrome and work organisation in repetitive work: a cross sectional study in France. Study Group on Repetitive *Work. Occup. Environ. Med.* (1998) 55: 180-187.

[19] Mondelli, M., Giannini, F., Giacchi, M. Carpal tunnel syndrome incidence in a general population. *Neurology* (2002) 58: 289-294.

[20] Nathan, P. A., Takigawa, K., Keniston, R. C., Meadows, K. D., Lockwood, R. S. Slowing of sensory conduction of the median nerve and carpal tunnel syndrome in Japanese and American industrial workers. *J. Hand Surg. Br.* (1994) 19: 30-34.

[21] Palmer, D. H., Hanrahan, L. P. Social and economic costs of carpal tunnel surgery. *Instr. Course Lect.* (1995) 44: 167-172.

[22] Palmer, K. T. Carpal tunnel syndrome: the role of occupational factors. *Best Pract. Res. Clin. Rheumatol.* (2011) 25: 15-29.

[23] Palmer, K. T., Harris, E. C., Coggon, D. Carpal tunnel syndrome and its relation to occupation: a systematic literature review. *Occup. Med.* (Lond.) (2007) 57: 57-66.

[24] Patil, V. S., Chopra, A. Watch out for 'pins and needles' in hands-it may be a case of gout. *Clin. Rheumatol.* (2007) 26: 2185-2187.

[25] Phalen, G. S. Spontaneous compression of the median nerve at the wrist. *J. Am. Med. Assoc.* (1951) 145: 1128-1133.

[26] Phalen, G. S., Gardner, W. J., La Londe, A. A. Neuropathy of the median nerve due to compression beneath the transverse carpal ligament. *J. Bone Joint Surg. Am.* (1950) 32A: 109-112.

[27] Phalen, G. S., Kendrick, J. I. Compression neuropathy of the median nerve in the carpal tunnel. *J. Am. Med. Assoc.* (1957) 164: 524-530.

[28] Pienimaki, T. Cold exposure and musculoskeletal disorders and diseases. A review. *Int. J. Circumpolar Health* (2002) 61: 173-182.

[29] Pourmemari, M. H., Viikari-Juntura, E., Shiri, R. Smoking and carpal tunnel syndrome: A meta-analysis. *Muscle Nerve* (2014) 49: 345-350.

[30] Raimbeau, G. [Recurrent carpal tunnel syndrome]. *Chir. Main* (2008) 27: 134-145.

[31] Rempel, D., Evanoff, B., Amadio, P. C., de Krom, M., Franklin, G., Franzblau, A., Gray, R., Gerr, F., Hagberg, M., Hales, T., Katz, J. N., Pransky, G. Consensus criteria for the classification of carpal tunnel syndrome in epidemiologic studies. *Am. J. Public Health* (1998) 88: 1447-1451.

[32] Roh, Y. H., Chung, M. S., Baek, G. H., Lee, Y. H., Rhee, S. H., Gong, H. S. Incidence of clinically diagnosed and surgically treated carpal tunnel syndrome in Korea. *J. Hand Surg. Am.* (2010) 35: 1410-1417.

[33] Rosenbaum, R. How should we assess quality of electrodiagnostic testing for carpal tunnel syndrome? *Muscle Nerve* (2010) 41: 439-440.

[34] Saeed, M. A., Irshad, M. Seasonal variation and demographical characteristics of carpal tunnel syndrome in a Pakistani population. *J. Coll. Physicians Surg. Pak.* (2010) 20: 798-801.

[35] Solomon, D. H., Katz, J. N., Bohn, R., Mogun, H., Avorn, J. Non-occupational risk factors for carpal tunnel syndrome. *J. Gen. Intern. Med.* (1999) 14: 310-314.

[36] Spahn, G., Wollny, J., Hartmann, B., Schiele, R., Hofmann, G. O. [Metaanalysis for the evaluation of risk factors for carpal tunnel syndrome (CTS) Part II. Occupational risk factors]. *Z. Orthop. Unfall.* (2012) 150: 516-524.

[37] Tanaka, S., Wild, D. K., Seligman, P. J., Behrens, V., Cameron, L., Putz-Anderson, V. The US prevalence of self-reported carpal tunnel syndrome: 1988 National Health Interview Survey data. *Am. J. Public Health* (1994) 84: 1846-1848.

[38] Thomsen, J. F., Gerr, F., Atroshi, I. Carpal tunnel syndrome and the use of computer mouse and keyboard: a systematic review. *BMC Musculo-skelet. Disord.* (2008) 9: 134.

[39] Tuppin, P., Blotiere, P. O., Weill, A., Ricordeau, P., Allemand, H. [Carpal tunnel syndrome surgery in France in 2008: patients' characteristics and management]. *Rev. Neurol.* (Paris) (2011) 167: 905-915.

[40] Van Meir, N., De Smet, L. Carpal tunnel syndrome in children. *Acta Orthop. Belg.* (2003) 69: 387-395.

[41] Viikari-Juntura, E., Silverstein, B. Role of physical load factors in carpal tunnel syndrome. *Scand. J. Work Environ. Health* (1999) 25: 163-185.

[42] Werner, R. A., Franzblau, A., Albers, J. W., Armstrong, T. J. Influence of body mass index and work activity on the prevalence of median mononeuropathy at the wrist. *Occup. Environ. Med.* (1997) 54: 268-271.

[43] Wessel, L. E., Fufa, D. T., Boyer, M. I., Calfee, R. P. Epidemiology of carpal tunnel syndrome in patients with single versus multiple trigger digits. *J. Hand Surg. Am.* (2013) 38: 49-55.

[44] Zyluk, A. Is carpal tunnel syndrome an occupational disease? A review. *Pol. Orthop. Traumatol.* (2013) 78: 121-126.

In: Carpal Tunnel Syndrome
Editor: Morton Ledford

ISBN: 978-1-63321-142-1
© 2014 Nova Science Publishers, Inc.

Chapter 8

Patient Reported Outcome Measures in Hand Surgery

Wasim S. Khan, Ph.D.[1,*] *and*
Matthew A. Ravenscroft, FRCS[2]

[1]University College London Institute of Orthopaedics
and Musculoskeletal Sciences, Royal National
Orthopaedic Hospital, Stanmore, London, UK
[2]Department of Trauma and Orthopaedics,
Stockport NHS Foundation Trust, Stepping
Hill Hospital, Stockport, UK

Abstract

Injuries and disease commonly affect the ability of an individual to perform activities of daily living. The use of regional outcome measures or scoring systems is important as it allows comparison between these injuries and disease, and allows clinicians to assess progression and the effects of different treatment modalities.

* Corresponding author: Mr. Wasim S. Khan, Academic Clinical Fellow, University College London Institute of Orthopaedics and Musculoskeletal Science, Royal National Orthopaedic Hospital, Stanmore, London, HA7 4LP, UK. Telephone number: +44 (0) 7971 190720, Fax number: +44 (0) 20 8570 3864, E-mail address: wasimkhan@doctors.org.uk.

A patient-completed questionnaire is efficient in terms of time and resources, and allows the assessment of outcome without the need to attend an outpatient clinic.

It is important that the scoring system allows satisfactory regional outcome measurements. The validity, reliability, responsiveness and bias are used for the assessment of various questionnaires.

There are also many practical issues concerning the use of questionnaires including feasibility of use for the patient and the clinician. This paper looks at why these measures should be used, their advantages and disadvantages, how they are developed and also how they should be presented. It aims to be useful to those who are developing new questionnaires, as well as those who are using them.

Why Use Regional Outcome Measures?

Injuries and disease commonly affect the hand as it is in regular use. Hand injuries alone account for almost a fifth of all accident and emergency department attendances. The last decade has seen a significant increase in different therapies, operative and non-operative in the management of diseases and injuries of the hand.

These injuries and disease are expensive and associated with increasing costs. This is because they can significantly affect the ability of an individual to perform activities of daily living, and have significant socio-economic consequences.

Direct costs of these injuries and disease are associated costs associated with the actual therapy. Indirect costs are those associated with the burden on the patient from time off work and lost income, and burden on the wider society from the loss of productivity.

The use of regional outcome measures or scoring systems is important as it not only allows comparison between these injuries and disease, but also allows clinicians to assess progression and the effects of different therapies (Currens, 2000). They are used in routine patient care, clinical audit and research, population surveys and epidemiological studies, resource allocation and assessing the quality of healthcare.

Regional outcome measures exist in many forms and allow the measure of outcome following injury, disease and therapy, and at various intervals. Over the last decade, there has been a shift in outcome measurements from objective measurements made by the clinician to subjective reporting by the patient. It allows a comparison to be made that would justify a change in therapy.

With a greater trend of measuring outcome to justify intervention, and its cost implications, it is likely that the use of regional outcome measures will continue to increase.

To identify the effect of these disease and injuries and the effect of various therapies, reliable and valid instruments are required to evaluate any differences. These instruments could also be used to predict the outcomes of different therapies. There is currently no standardised or universally accepted evaluation instrument for the hand (Bucher and Hume, 2002). Although goniometers and dynamometers are routinely used in clinical practice, they only assess structure and function. There is no standard instrument to assess limitation of activities in patients with limited hand function.

Questionnaires as Regional Outcome Measures

The use of questionnaires for data collection in hand surgery, and in all other healthcare disciplines has increased in recent years. Questionnaires allow the collection of data in a standardised manner. With increasing emphasis on evidence-based practice, it is becoming increasingly important to collect data on injuries and disease, and evaluate the effectiveness of various therapies.

Questionnaires consist of a series of questions or statements that the patients respond to. These responses are then converted to numeral form and statistically analysed.

Questionnaires have many advantages over other regional outcome measures. They take little time to complete, have fewer associated costs and are generally easy to analyse (Bowling, 1997).

Patient-completed disease-specific questionnaires for the hand include the Australian/Canadian Osteoarthritis (AUSCAN) Hand Index.

Regional outcome measures are relevant to potentially all pathologies within that region, unlike disease-specific questionnaires that are only relevant to a particular pathology.

Although disease-specific questionnaires are more responsive due to the focussed questions, they are limited in their applicability to only a single disorder.

There Patient Outcome of Surgery- Hand/ Arm (POS-Hand/ Arm) is not a disease-specific questionnaire, but for evaluating outcomes in surgery for hand and arm disorders (Cano et al., 2004). It has a greater scope than disease-specific questionnaires but it nevertheless is limited compared to other regional outcome measures as it cannot be used in certain circumstances.

A large number of hand diseases and injuries are managed non-operatively making the POS-Hand/ Arm irrelevant. It would also not be applicable when trying to ascertain the impact of physiotherapy. Furthermore the developers of the questionnaire designed it with the aim of specifically targeting elective non-malignant surgery.

Why Use Patient-Completed Questionnaires?

Patient-completed questionnaires are being increasingly favoured in medical research although there is little evidence to suggest that they are more valid than clinician-completed questionnaires.

Patient-completed questionnaires have many advantages over clinician-completed questionnaires. One of the most important factors is cost. Patient-completed questionnaires save time as they can be completed by the patient in the waiting room or at home.

The clinician-completed questionnaire on the other hand takes time away from the clinician, and slows down the consultation and the clinic. Telephone questionnaires do reduce the costs associated with clinician-completed questionnaires but they do not negate many of the other disadvantages. In a study comparing the results of health surveys, it was noted that patients were more likely to report health problems in patient-completed questionnaires than in clinician-completed questionnaires (Cook et al., 1993).

Clinician-completed questionnaires can be useful as they can result in a higher response rate and fewer omissions from the questionnaire. They may result in a more thorough consultation, and more information and clarification on particular questions can be made available to the patient. This however may not always be the case as the questionnaire may not be completed by the clinician or the clinician looking after the patient, particularly in blinded studies. Patient-completed questionnaires, by virtue of their design, aim to be clear and concise avoiding the need for further explanation by the clinician.

Patient-completed questionnaires also have the advantage of letting the patient complete the questionnaire at their leisure, and they do not feel rushed into providing just any answer. They do not result in answer bias that could be a feature in clinician-completed questionnaires if the clinician conducting the questionnaire has not received the relevant training to use the questionnaire.

Postal questionnaires are cheaper than interview or telephone completed questionnaires, and evidence suggests that patients are more likely to report poorer health states.

Why Use Fixed-Response Questions?

The responses for the questions in the patient-completed questionnaires could be in many formats. Fixed-response questions are generally preferred as they allow categorisation of the response. There are many types of scales that are available including the frequency scales, Thurstone scales, Guttman scales and Likert scales. Frequency scales are numerical and establish how often an event occurs. Thurston scales use empirical data to ensure clinical features being measured are spaced along a continuum. Gutman scales are hierarchical where a higher category response suggests agreement with all lower category responses. Likert scales assume a linear response and a choice of four to nine responses are available between on a continuum from strongly agree to strongly disagree.

At one extreme, only two possible responses exist. At the other extreme, the patients may be presented with a line and chose a response between two extremes i.e. the visual analogue scale. The two possible responses can be frustrating for the patient who fail to better express themselves, and are not much use to the clinician as they do not provide any additional information to enable a more thorough assessment.

These two extremes have been falling out of favour and now there is a greater tendency to provide patients with between four and nine fixed responses to choose from. In a study, a seven fixed-response questionnaire was found to be as responsive as the visual analogue score, and easier to administer and interpret. The data generates scores that are used as interval data and allow the use of parametric tests.

It is important however that the fixed responses are logical, avoid overlap and cover the likely response range. There is potential to skew data if the likely response range is not covered appropriately within the categories. There is controversy regarding the provision of a neutral point, as if it was removed it would force the patient to choose a response.

Close-Ended and Open-Ended Questions

Questionnaires usually comprise of closed questions. Open-ended questions may allow the patient to express themselves better, but are difficult for clinicians to analyse. The responses tend to be highly subjective and may not address the issues that the questionnaire wants to address.

It is unusual however to see questionnaires with only open-ended questions, and many questionnaires have fixed-response questions with the option of an open-ended question at the end.

In such cases it can be useful for the patient by allowing them to better express themselves. They also allow the expression of concerns that would have been brought up in a consultation during a clinician-completed questionnaire.

It also allows the clinician to gain insight into the patients' responses. The open-ended questions have an important role in the developing of a questionnaire, but not particularly so in a well-developed questionnaire.

Why Use Domains with More Than One Question?

Domains are areas of interest that are covered by the questionnaire. In hand questionnaires they tend to be pain, function etc. In many questionnaires there are predetermined domains e.g. pain, function etc., and one or more questions for each domain.

It is usual to have more than one question for each domain as it allows a more thorough assessment of each domain. They reduce bias, misinterpretation and reduce measurement error, and they have been shown to be more reliable (Streiner and Norman, 1994).

Symptoms like pain and function are complex and multifaceted, and one question alone is generally insufficient to satisfactorily assess them.

A number of questions would allow a more thorough assessment of the domain and reduce the chances of bias due to a single answer. It is however important that all questions within the domain are relevant to that domain and are internally consistent.

In the creation of questionnaires first domains are identified and likely questions for each domain are gathered. This is done in a variety of ways. It is commonly done by conducting interviews with patient groups, with an expert panel of clinicians or both.

It could also be done by a literature review. This results in a number of questions, some of which may be redundant. Pilot studies are performed where some of the questions are eliminated by statistical factor analyses.

Development of a Questionnaire

There are international guidelines (Scientific Advisory Committee of the Medical Outcome Trust, 2002) for the development and validation of health outcome measure questionnaires. The guidelines describe a rigorous, three-stage, gold standard methodology. It briefly comprises of three stages. In the first stage, a pool of items is generated from interviews with patient interviews and experts, and a review of the literature. This results in the development of a conceptual model. In the second stage, the large pool of items is field tested by postal survey to select questions that showed the best scientific performance. Scales are also identified at this stage. In the third stage the measurement properties of the new measure are further tested by a further postal survey of an independent group of patients.

The first stage in the development of a questionnaire is item generation that usually encompasses a number of domains. A comprehensive selection of questions is identified along with responses that cover all aspects of the disease. This is done through patient and clinician interviews and review of the literature. This is followed by item reduction following a field test of the questionnaire where the number of questions is reduced to a reasonable size by removing unnecessary and repetitive questions. This also relies on expert opinion and statistical analyses to determine the redundancy of a question, its endorsement frequency and factor analyses. Missing data is also assessed to identify any trends and determine the cause for it and questions may need to be rephrases or removed.

This is followed by pilot studies and psychometric analyses. This allows the performance and relevance of the questions and the questionnaire as a whole to be assessed. Questions are then be statistically analysed to assess their validity and reliability before they are eliminated or rephrased. Pilot studies allow a trial of the questionnaire using a sample population that the questionnaire would ultimately be targeted at. The completed questionnaires are then statistically analysed to assess the acceptability, validity, internal consistency, item total correlation, reliability, responsiveness, bias and range.

The validity establishes whether the outcome measure actually measures what it was designed to. The criterion, construct, and content or face validity provide various assessment parameters that allow a complete picture of the validity of a questionnaire to be established. An outcome tool has test-retest reproducibility if the same result is obtained when tested at different time points once the condition has stabilised. The responsiveness is the ability to detect clinically important changes in disability at various intervals.

The effect size and the standardised response mean are used to evaluate the responsiveness. Bias can occur when assumed independent variables such as age, gender, hand dominance or dominant side injured affect responses.

In general, if there is more than 5% missing data for a particular question, it should be rephrased or removed. The endorsement frequency i.e. the proportion of respondents who endorse a particular response category, is also important. The endorsement frequency should be between 20% and 80%.

If the endorsement frequency is outside this range, it suggests that there is inadequate spread of response categories.

If a response for a particular question is chosen very often or not often enough, it suggests that the response has poor discriminatory power and that it is redundant and can be excluded.

In general there are two easy ways of analysing a pilot questionnaire. Item analysis is often used in pilot studies to decide if a question or response should be retained or deleted. High endorsement of a response option suggests poor discriminatory power and should be deleted. An alternative method is to use the Cronbach's alpha. This is used to show that the questionnaire measures a single construct and that questions can be combined to form a summary score. Cronbach's alpha coefficients for summary scores should be greater 0.70. A lower value suggests that the questions in the questionnaire are poorly grouped. It is important that individual questions measure distinct but related constructs. Item–total correlations for individual questions should have a value of greater than 0.30, and questions that have a value of less than 0.30 are assumed not to add to the value of the questionnaire and should be excluded.

However, despite the above analyses, it is important to bear in mind the original questionnaire and the theoretical domains, as these may sometimes overrule any poor statistical performance. Pilot studies are performed that aim to identify any potential problems with questionnaires so that they could be dealt with before the formal use of a questionnaire. Pilot studies can identify questions frequently omitted and look at the cause that may be inappropriate wording of a question. Pilot studies also allow the refining of words and content. Often open-ended questions are introduced only in pilot studies so further information and feedback from the questionnaire could be obtained.

Presentation of the Questionnaire

The way a questionnaire is presented is vital. A well-structured questionnaire following a logical order that is easy to follow will result in a high response rate and have fewer omissions. It is important that there are clear explanations to the patients, often in the form of an accompanying letter, detailing the purpose of the questionnaire, why the patient has been asked to complete the questionnaire, and clear instructions on how to complete the questionnaire.

If open-ended questions are being used, it is important that there is enough space available for a response. It is important that the questionnaire is well-laid out, uses polite language and the text is readable. The order of the questions is also important and any optional questions should be included at the end of the questionnaires. Controversial and emotive questions should ideally be placed towards the end of the questionnaire.

It is also worth arranging the questions with a mixture of positively and negatively worded questions to minimise acquiescent response bias. Although many of these statements are common sense, they can easily be overlooked in the difficult technicalities of developing the questionnaire.

The Ideal Patient-Completed Questionnaire

The ideal patient-completed questionnaire for outcome assessment of the hand, or indeed any outcome assessment, does not exist. The ideal questionnaire should enable the patient to convey the relevant information, and for the clinician to satisfactorily use that information.

For this to happen, both the patient and the clinician need to be thought of when designing a questionnaire.

The questionnaire, as it is to be completed by the patient, should avoid technical terms as these may not be understood, or worse, misunderstood by the patient.

They should avoid ambiguity and bias, and use simple short phrases. It is important to avoid 'double barrelled' questions, and 'double negative' questions. By making the questionnaire more acceptable to the patient, there should be a higher response rate and fewer omissions in the questionnaires.

It is also important that any questionnaire puts minimum burden on the rater or respondent in terms of time and effort to ensure optimal compliance. It should not place any financial burden on the respondent and postage should be paid for by the physician or researcher.

It is also important that any questionnaire puts minimum administrative burden on the physician or researcher in terms of extracting information from the questionnaire, inputting data on a database and calculating the score.

Conclusion

This paper aims to provide some basic information regarding questionnaires and an overall assessment of the practicalities and statistical analyses. The choice of instrument to be used will depend on many factors including the project, population and setting, mode of administration, and time and financial constraints.

References

Atroshi, I., Gummesson, C., Johnsson, R., Sprinchorn, A. (1999). Symptoms, disability and quality of life in patients with carpal tunnel syndrome. *J. Hand Surg*. 24A: 398-404.

Baldry Currens, J. A. (2000). Evaluation of disability and handicap following injury. *Injury*. 31: 99-106.

Bowling, A. (1997). *Research Methods in Health*. Open University Press, Buckingham.

Cano, S. J., Browne, J. P., Lamping, D. L., Roberts, A. H., McGrouther, D. A., Black, N. A. (2004). The Patient Outcomes of Surgery-Hand/Arm (POS-Hand/Arm): a new patient-based outcome measure. *J. Hand Surg*. 29: 477-485.

Cook, D., Guyatt, G., Juniper, E., Griffith, L., McIlroy, W., Willan, A., Jaeschke, R., Epstein, R. (1993). Interviewer versus self-administered questionnaires in developing health-related quality of life instrument for asthma. *J. Clin. Epidem.* 46: 529-534.

Guyatt, G., Townsend, M., Berman, L., Keller, J. (1987). A comparison of Likert and visual analogue scales for measuring change in function. *J. Chron. Dis.* 40: 1229-1233.

Khan, W., Jain, R., Dillon, B., Clarke, L., Fehily, M., Ravenscroft, M. (2008). The 'M2 DASH'-Manchester-modified Disabilities of Arm Shoulder and Hand score. *Hand* (NY). 3: 240-244.

Khan, W., Dillon, B., Agarwal, M., Fehily, M., Ravenscroft, M. (2009). The validity, reliability, responsiveness and bias of the Manchester-Modified Disabilities of Arm Shoulder and Hand score in hand injuries. *Hand* (NY) (in press).

MacDermid, J. C., Richards, R. S., Donner, A., Bellamy, N., Roth, J. H. (2000). Responsiveness of the short form-36, disability of the arm, shoulder, and hand questionnaire, patient-rated wrist evaluation, and physical impairment measurements in evaluating recovery after a distal radius fracture. *J. Hand Surg.* 25A: 330-340.

Macey, A. C., Burke, F. D., Abbott, K., Barton, N. J., Bradbury, E., Bradley, A., Bradley, M. J., Brady, O., Burt, A., Brown, P. (1995). Outcomes of hand surgery. British Society for Surgery of the Hand. *J. Hand Surg.* 20B: 841-855.

Streiner, D., Norman, G. (1994). *Health Measurement Scales*. Oxford: Oxford University Press.

Wood-Dauphinee, S. (1999). Assessing quality of life in clinical research: from where have we come and where are we going? *J. Clin. Epidemiol.* 52: 355-363.

Reviewed by: Mr. Manish Agarwal, FRCS (Orth), Department of Trauma and Orthopaedics, Pennine Acute Hospitals NHS Trust, North Manchester General Hospital, Manchester, M8 5RB, UK.

In: Carpal Tunnel Syndrome
Editor: Morton Ledford

ISBN: 978-1-63321-142-1
© 2014 Nova Science Publishers, Inc.

Chapter 9

Carpal Tunnel Syndrome: Carpal Tunnel Release – Mini-Open Technique

Sergio Gennaro[1], M.D., Pietro Fiaschi[1]*, M.D. and Paolo Merciadri[1], M.D.

[1]Department of Neurosurgery, San Martino, IST University Hospital (IRCCS), Genoa, Italy

Abstract

Carpal tunnel syndrome (CTS) is a common disorder in hand surgery practice. Both surgical and conservative interventions are utilized for the carpal tunnel syndrome, although certain indications would specifically indicate the need for surgery.

Conservative management is typically preferred for transient cases of CTS such as those associated with pregnancy, short-term overuse or where other exacerbating phenomena are expected to be corrected. In other cases conservative management might be used for partial relief of symptoms while awaiting surgery or for diagnostic purposes in determining patient response [1].

* Corresponding author: Pietro Fiaschi, M.D.; Department of Neurosurgery, San Martino - IST University Hospital (IRCCS), Largo Rosanna Benzi 10, 16132 Genoa, Italy. Phone +39.3402767717; email: pietro.fiaschi@alice.it.

The surgical intervention for CTS is recommended in remaining case, in which is common to find out these characteristics: constant numbness, symptoms > 1 year durations, sensory loss, thenar weakness/atrophy.

The first popularization of diagnosis and treatment of "carpal tunnel syndrome" is attributed to Phalen in 1950. Since then, there has been continued debate over the optimal management of this disease [2]. Currently, surgical options include these techniques: carpal tunnel release with a standard open, carpal tunnel release using various incision techniques (such as mini-open), endoscopic carpal tunnel release, open carpal tunnel release with additional procedures such as internal neurolysis, epineurotomy or tenosynovectomy.

From August 2004 to November 2013, 780 procedures of carpal tunnel release using a mini open incision technique have been performed in our department.

The procedure starts with an accurate skin detersion and disinfection. The intervention has been performed under local anesthesia and exsanguination with pneumatic tourniquet at the limb. The wrist extended approximately 30°. 2 cm long scalpel incision on Taleisnik line. Retraction of skin edges, incision of palmar aponeurosis, exposition and complete opening of flexor retinaculum to perform an external neurolysis of median nerve from fibro/adherential tissue. Before the wound closure a water dissection is performed to complete the procedure and to evaluate the decompression within the carpal tunnel.

Postoperative bulky dressing and skin sutures are kept for 10 days and then removed.

No complications like nerve, vascular or tendon damage, nor infection, relapse or failed treatment occurred. The one exception was a case of postoperative wound infection in a patient who dirtied the dressing during activities in a farm. In all cases patients referred a fast total regression of preoperatively symptoms. No painful and hypertrophic scars were observed.

Introduction

In our opinion, the surgical procedure starts when the patient enters the operating room. The professional and kind behavior of the health workers and the monitoring of blood pressure, ECG and pulse oximetry, immediately impart self-confidence and reassurance to the patient and on the other hand are essential tools for a safe procedure.

The procedure can be divided in three different steps, each one important in preventing possible complications:

1) positioning of the patient on the operating table
2) skin disinfection and preparation of the surgical field
3) surgical intervention

Procedure

1) Patient Positioning

The patient is placed in supine position with the head raised to 30 degrees in order to grant an optimal respiratory function (Figure 1). The upper art is comfortably abducted to 80-90 degrees and the radiocarpal joint is slightly extended to push the medial nerve in a more superficial position and to maintain the palmar surface and the flexor retinaculum parallel to the floor. This position helps to perform an orthogonal transection of the flexor retinaculum (and to avoid an ineffective "beveled angle" incision).

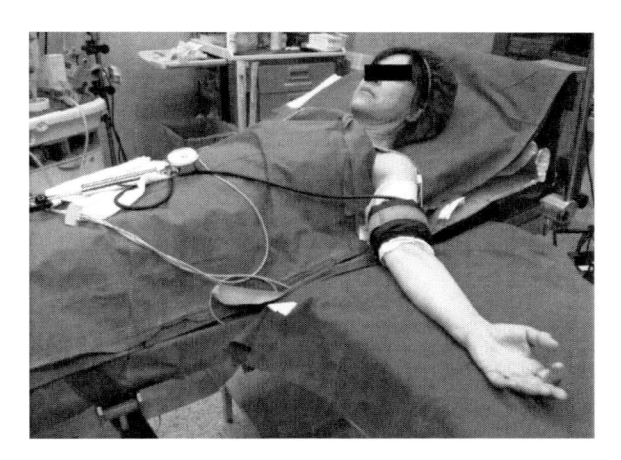

Figure 1. Positioning of the Patient.

2) Skin Disinfection and Preparation of the Surgical Field

Once the correct position of the patient on the operating table is checked, the pneumatic tourniquet is positioned to maintain a bloodless surgical field. The skin is then carefully brushed using the same kind of brush/sponge usually used by the surgeon himself for the surgical hand scrub (Figure 2). The sponge is impregnated povidone-iodine solution (7.5%). This solution is rinsed out with normal saline and finally the disinfection is concluded using an alcoholic solution (benzalkonium chloride 0,25% and ethylic alcohol 70%). The entire brushing/disinfecting procedure takes about three minutes to be completed (Figure 3, Figure 4).

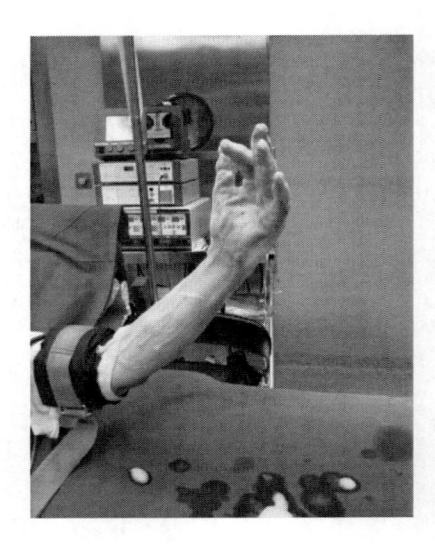

Figure 2. Skin disinfection.

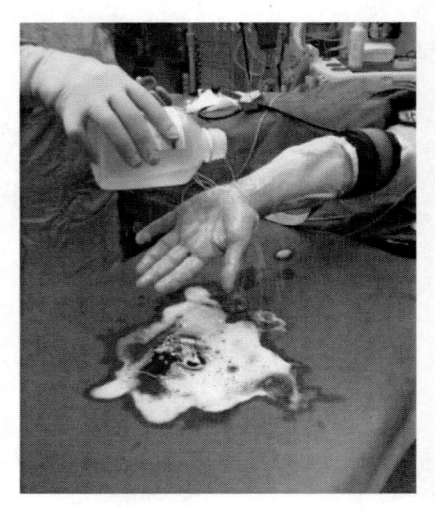

Figure 3. Skin disinfection.

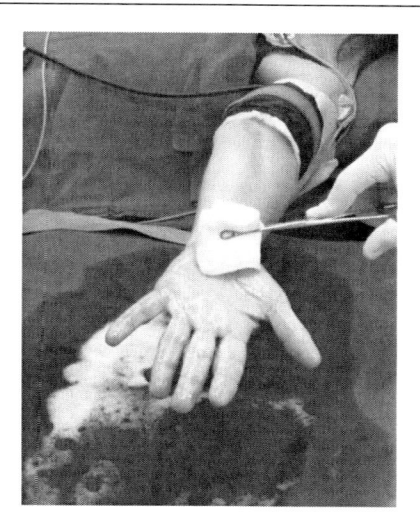

Figure 4. Skin disinfection.

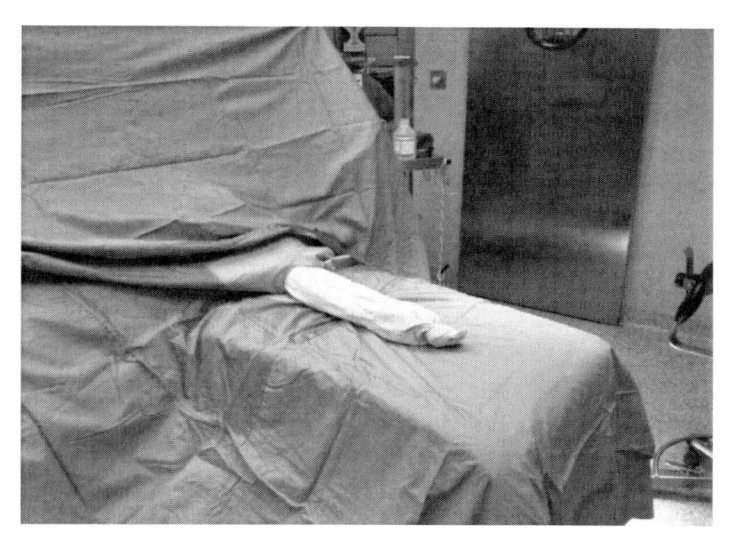

Figure 5. Preparation of the surgical field.

Once the surgical field is prepared (Figure 5), the surgeon injects 3-4 cubic centimeters of mepivacaine hydrochloride 1% and sodium bicarbonate on the palm of the hand, medially to the thenar eminence and distally to the wrist crease (Figure 6).

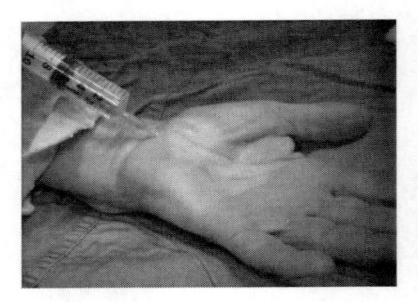

Figure 6. Local anesthesia.

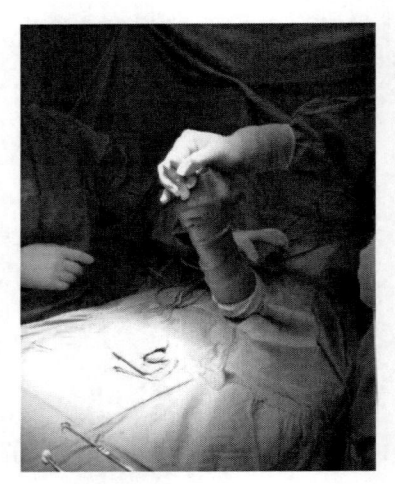

Figure 7. Forearm ischemia.

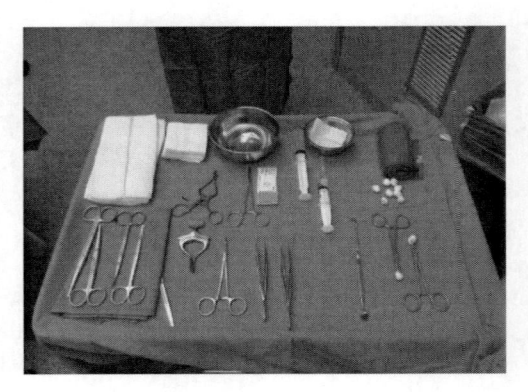

Figure 8. Surgical instrumentation.

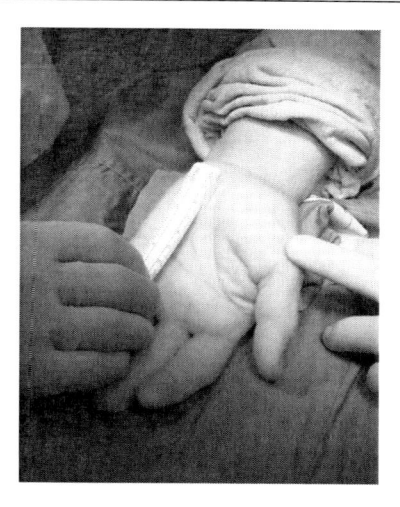

Figure 9. Skin incision.

The ischemia is obtained wrapping the Esmarch bandage around the arm and inflating the pneumatic tourniquet to a pressure about 100 mmHg higher than the systemic blood pressure (Figure 7).

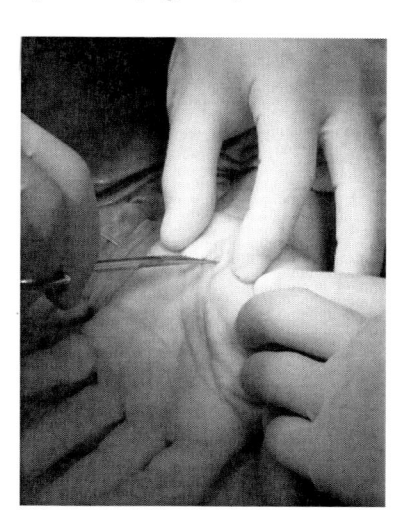

Figure 10. Superficial layers dissection.

3) Surgical Intervention

- *Skin incision:* a 20 millimeters linear skin incision is performed in the most proximal part of the palm of the hand along the extension of the line of Taleisnik immediately distally to the wrist crease (Figure 8, Figure 9, Figure 10)

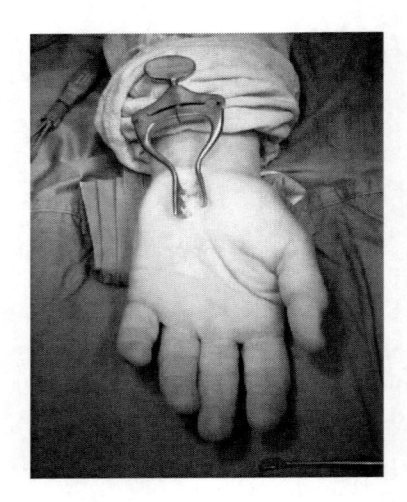

Figure 11. Flexor retinaculum exposure.

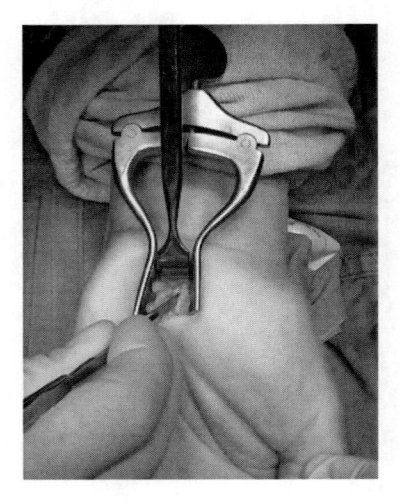

Figure 12. Flexor retinaculum opening.

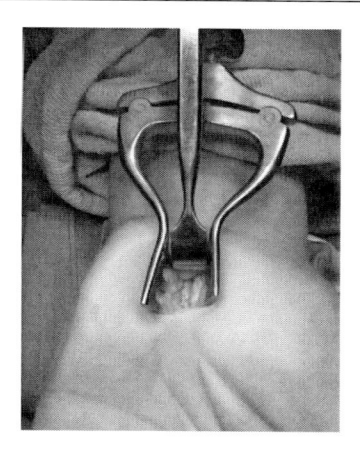

Figure 13. Reticulotomy.

- *Flexor retinaculum exposure (Figure 11):* with the dissecting scissors, the fibers of the palmar aponeurosis are opened. A small superficial retractor is inserted and the flexor retinaculum is exposed.

- *Flexor retinaculum opening (Figure 12)*: when performing reticulotomy between the bellies of the opponent muscles of the first and fifth fingers of the hand, initially a small breach in the middle third of the retinaculum is realized, then with blunt scissors the opening in its distal segment is completed, until displaing of adipose palmar tissue, subsequently in its proximal segment, lifting with a small retractor the skin and the fibers of the aponeurosis (Figure 13).

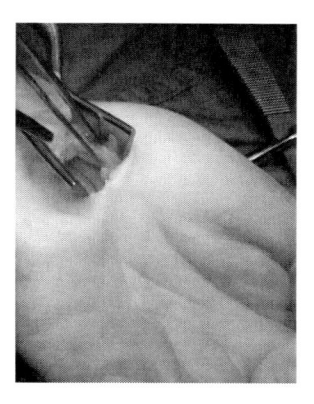

Figure 14. Median nerve visualization.

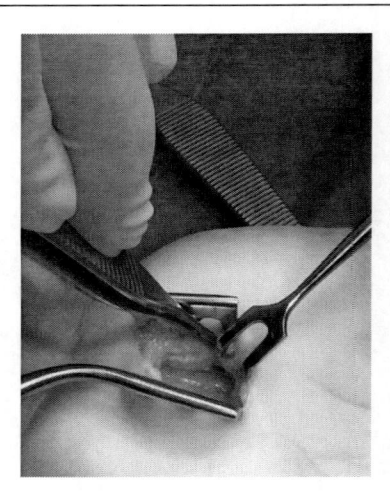

Figure 15. External neurolysis with exposition of I motor.

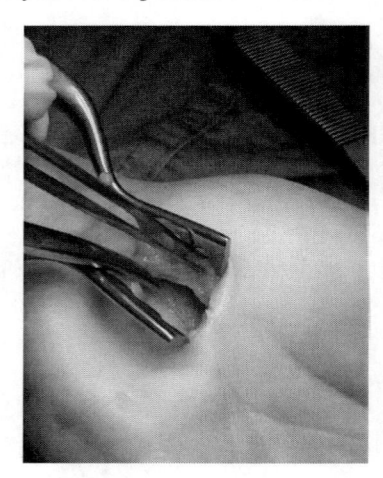

Figure 16. Early epineural rivascularization.

- *External neurolysis of the median nerve:* after reticulotomy is performed, raising with an Adson surgical forceps the radial margin of flexor retinaculum, you can see the rapid resumption of epineural revascularization on the volar side of the nerve (Figure 14, Figure 15, Figure 16). However in this phase of intervention, through repeated flexion-extension movement of the fingers actively produced by the patient, an indirect trauma on the nerve is still detectable, related to synovial tight adhesions that "anchor" the nerve to the underlying flexor tendons.

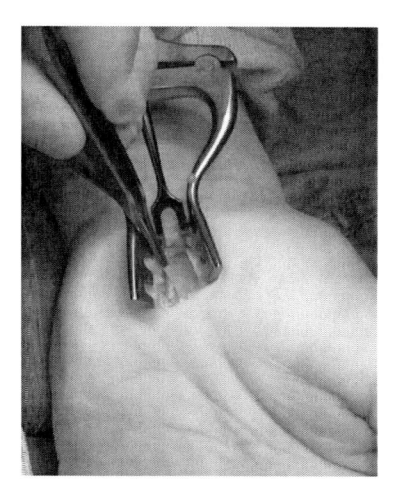

Figure 17. Sinovial tissue removal.

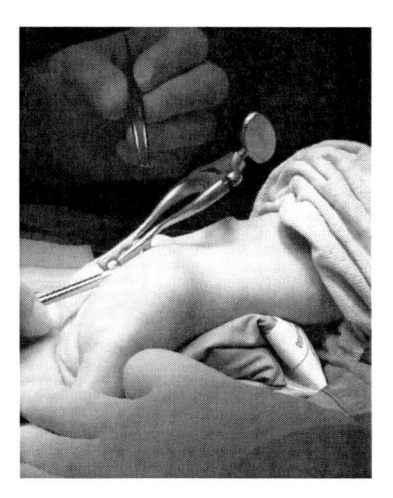

Figure 18. Complete proximal opening check.

It is therefore indispensable, in addition to the complete opening of flexor retinaculum, even the rupture of synovial adhesions on the nerve at 360 degrees, in order to resolve this conflict. In compressive forms, when you should encounter an abundant reactive synovial tissue, it is recommended for removal.

After completing the external neurolysis on the radial side, the first motor branch of the median nerve with the flexor tendons of the first finger are visible, and you can still see how the flexion-extension movement of the fingers no more will result in an indirect trauma on the nerve. Median nerve also will tend to radialization with a more physiological course, protected by the muscle belly of the opponent and by the radial margin of the retinaculum (Figure 18).

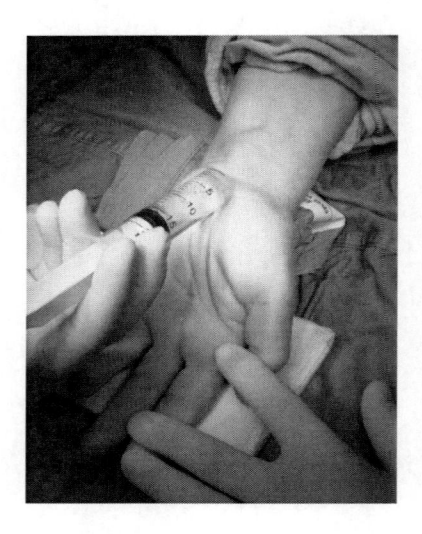

Figure 19. Proximal water dissection.

Water Dissection

In the proximal and distal part of surgical exposure, in order to reduce nervous morbidity, synovial dissection is completed infusing with a syringe 8-10 cc of pressurized physiological solution (Figure 19, Figure 20).

Wound Closure

After performing a scrupulous hemostasis and monitoring the physiological revascularization of the limb, the skin is closed with separate points and without the placement of a drainage (Figure 21).

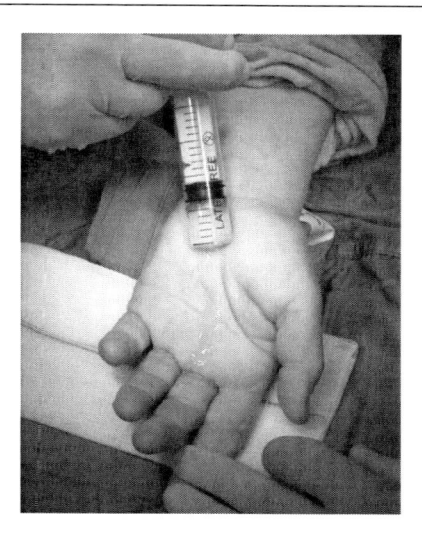

Figure 20. Distal water dissection.

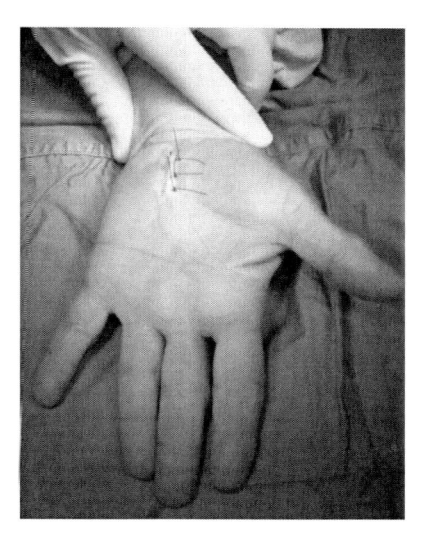

Figure 21. Wound closure and hand rivascularization.

Medication

After suturing the skin, on the surgical wound is placed a small gauze soaked with hydrogen peroxide and initially packaged with a cotton bandage then with an adhesive elastic bandage, finally, a handheld bandage with attitude of the wrist in slight flexion (Figure 22, Figure 23).

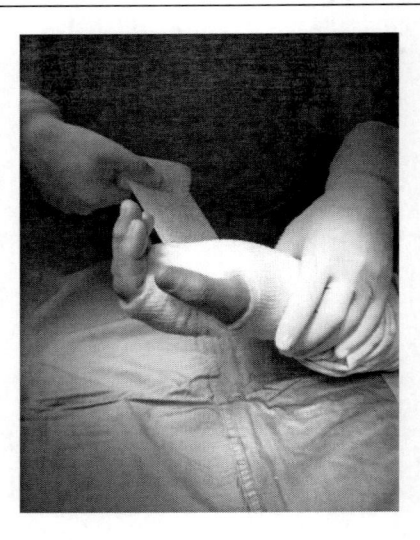

Figure 22. Dressing preparation.

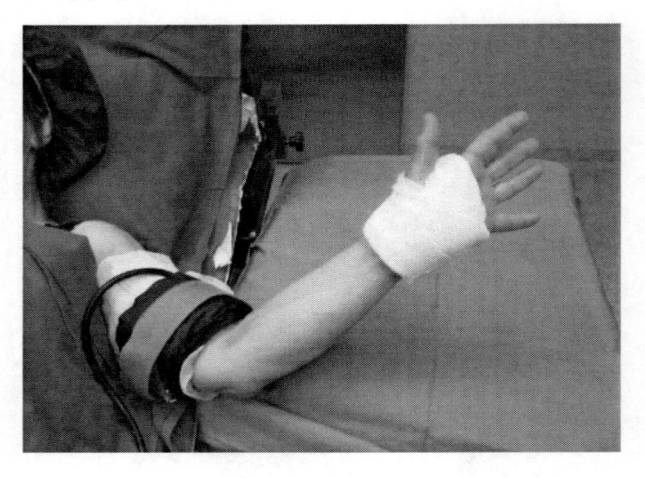

Figure 23. Final Result.

Conclusion

When the health professionals involved are in harmony, surgeons experience routine and scrupulous execution of all phases of the intervent that can be realized with the "mini-open" surgical technique, achieving Median nerve decompression in about 8 minutes.

This method also allows the surgeon to explore the median nerve under continuous visual control, to identify the many possible nervous anatomical variants, to highlight the rare but possible palmar neoformations responsible for compressive neuropathy and consequently to minimize the possible iatrogenic -infectious complications.

In: Carpal Tunnel Syndrome
Editor: Morton Ledford

ISBN: 978-1-63321-142-1
© 2014 Nova Science Publishers, Inc.

Chapter 10

Understanding Median Nerve Entrapment at the Wrist: Surgeon's Perspective of Carpal Tunnel Syndrome

*Moon Seok Kim and Jae Taek Hong**
Department of Neurosurgery, Catholic University of Korea,
St. Vincent's Hospital, Suwon, South Korea

Abstract

Since Sir James Paget firstly described carpal tunnel syndrome (CTS) in 1854, CTS has been reported the most common compressive neuropathy of the upper extremity. In 1933, Learmonth published firstly surgical release of the transverse carpal ligament by blind surgical treatment and in 1946, Cannon et al. performed the carpal tunnel release for spontaneous CTS firstly. Since then, diagnosis and treatment in CTS has much progressed. Currently, carpal tunnel decompression is the most common operation for peripheral nerves, with more than 586,000 procedures performed in the United States (US), 2006 alone.

* Corresponding Author: Jae Taek Hong, M.D. Professor; Address: 442-723, 93-6 Ji-Dong, Paldal-Gu, Suwon, Kyounggi-do, Korea; St. Vincent's Hospital, Catholic University of Korea; Tel : +82-31- 249-7190; Fax : +82-31-245-5208; E-mail: jatagi15@gmail.com

The prevalence of clinically and electrophysiologically confirmed CTS is 2.7% (approximately 3% in women and 2% in men) with peak prevalence in women of 55 to 64 years. A few studies have estimated the incidence of CTS, showing large differences between countries. The annual incidence was 324 in women and 125 in men per 100 000 persons in the general population in southern Sweden, and 542 in women and 304 in men per 100,000 persons in the US. In Korea, total clinically and electrophysiologically diagnosed CTS patients were 4.96 and 0.98 per 1,000 person-years, respectively.

The pathophysiology of CTS is associated with compression of the median nerve arising from increased pressure within the carpal tunnel. Incompatibility between decreased space in the carpal tunnel and increased volume of carpal tunnel contents may result in CTS.

CTS can be diagnosed on the basis of patient's history and clinical findings. Some physical examinations are important, but not exclusive for a CTS diagnosis. Advances in scientific tools such as neurophysiological test, MRI and ultrasonography are much helpful in diagnosis, also provided valuable insights into the pathophysiology of CTS.

Treatment of CTS may be selected considering the stage of the disease, the severity of the symptoms, or the preference of the patient. If conservative treatment failed, surgery should be considered, such as conventional open carpal tunnel release (OCTR), mini-OTCR, and endoscopic carpal tunnel release (ETCR).

There has been a variety of surgical techniques for the operative treatment of carpal tunnel syndrome (CTS). Recently, minimally invasive techniques for decompression of the median nerve were developed and introduced such as endoscopic carpal tunnel release (ECTR) and use of a carpal tunnel tome with a small palmar incision. Although many investigators described the advantages of minimally invasive carpal tunnel decompression techniques, numerous cases of iatrogenic injury to the neurovascular structure have been reported. Insufficient anatomical understanding of the carpal tunnel and poor visualization of the surgical field are two major causes of complication during minimally invasive surgery for CTS. In addition, hematoma formation associated with carpal tunnel release may lead to an increased rate of wound infection or delay in wound healing.

To obtain a good surgical outcome for CTS, it is essential to understand the neurovascular anatomy and anatomic variation around the carpal tunnel that these neurovascular structures may take. This chapter will also discuss the anatomical variations and about the changing location of the neurovascular structures during various wrist positions, especially since the wrist position can change unintentionally during surgery using local anesthesia.

History

Carpal tunnel syndrome (CTS), described by Paget in 1854, is the most frequent compressive peripheral neuropathy resulted from the compression of the median nerve at the wrist beneath the transverse carpal ligament [1, 2]. During the first half of the 20th century, however, most patients with carpal tunnel syndrome were diagnosed as having compression of either the brachial plexus or thenar nerve motor branch of the median nerve. In 1933, Learmonth published firstly surgical release of the transverse carpal ligament by blind surgical treatment. The first definitive surgical procedure was described and published by Canon et al. in 1946 [3, 4].

Phalen et al. coined the term "carpal tunnel syndrome in 1950 [5, 6]. As late as 1950, only twelve patients with operative release of the transverse carpal ligament for idiopathic carpal tunnel syndrome had been reported. Since 1960, CTS has become the most frequently diagnosed of peripheral compression-induced neuropathies [7].

Anatomy

Knowledge of normal and variant anatomy is fundamental not only to understand the pathophysiology of the carpal tunnel syndrome but also to avoid nerve injury during wrist surgery. The median nerve is a mixed motor and sensory nerve. The sensory distribution is from the radial three and a half digits and a part of the thenar eminence. The motor supply is to the first two lumbrical and to the thenar eminence muscles. The median nerve normally divides into six branches at the distal terminus of the flexor retinaculum.

The carpal tunnel is a well-defined, inelastic channel located in the volar wrist [8-11]. It is oval in shape and extends from the distal volar wrist crease to the mid-palm, just proximal to the superficial palmar arch. The carpal tunnel is bordered ulnarly by the hook of the hamate, triquetrum, and pisiform, radially by the trapezium, scaphoid, and flexor carpi radialis retinaculum, dorsally by the concave arch of the carpal bones and metacarpa lbases of the central rays, and anteriorly by the transverse carpal ligament (TCL) (Figure 1). The TCL measures 1 to 3 mm in thickness throughout its length about 4 to 6 cm and is 3 to 4 cm wide. The size of the carpal tunnel is about the size of the index finger in diameter, and the flexor tendons and median nerve glide past each other with ease within the carpal tunnel when it is of sufficient size.

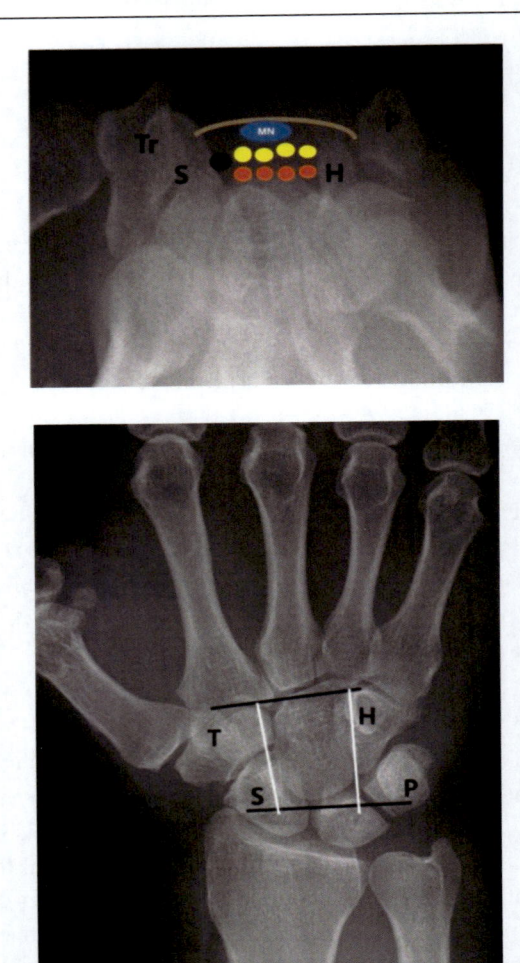

Figure 1. A) Drawing of in the carpal tunnel view shows the bony boundary and the contents in the carpal tunnel. The location of the median nerve (MN) is superficial to the tendons of flexor digitorum muscles and flexor policislongus muscle. B) Drawing in the wrist AP image shows the boundary of the carpal tunnel. Carpal tunnel is defined by 4 bony prominences; proximally, by pisiform& tubercle of scaphoid; distally by hook of hamate& tubercle of trapezium; from hamate & pisiform medially to scaphoid & trapezium laterally Tr; Trapezium, P; Pysiform, H; Hook of hamate, S; Scaphoid.

But in such a small, confined space, especially if it is not stable or is collapsing due to a lack of extensor/abductor muscle strength supporting the carpal bones, the median nerve can become impinged by the collapsing structures, and over time, severely damage the function of the median nerve. If the tendon size increases due to inflammation or hypertrophy, or if the carpal tunnel size decreases in size due to laxity in the joint, the structures within the carpal tunnel become impinged and carpal tunnel syndrome results.

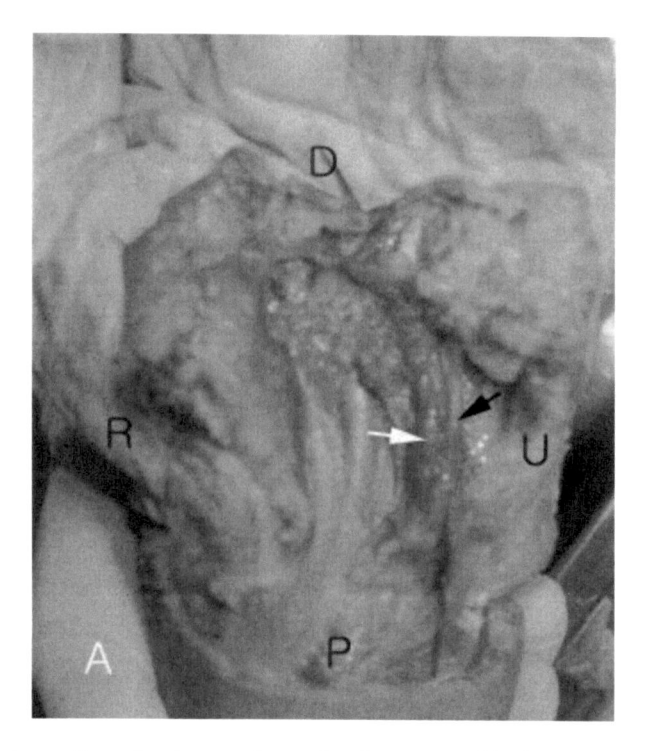

Figure 2. Cadaver dissection image shows the ulnar nerve (black arrow) and artery (white arrow) located close to the carpal tunnel and run superficially on the ulnar side of the TCL. P; proximal, D; distal, R; radial, U; ulnar.

Carpal tunnel lies deep to palmaris longus and the median nerve in the wrist is located superficially beneath the flexor retinaculum. Through this narrow osteofibrous tunnel, the median nerve is vulnerable to compression as it passes with the flexor pollicis longus and the eight flexor digitorum tendons. The ulnar nerve and artery run superficially on the ulnar side of the TCL, and the tendon of the flexor carpi radialis is enveloped by two layers of the TCL on the radial side of the wrist (Figure 2).

The finger / wrist flexor muscles and their tendons originate in the forearm at the medial epicondyle of the elbow joint and attach to the Metacarpal bones and first phalange (MP joint) and the first phalange and second phalange (PIP joint) and the second phalange and the third phalange (except for the thumb), which make up the distal (DIP) joint [12, 13].

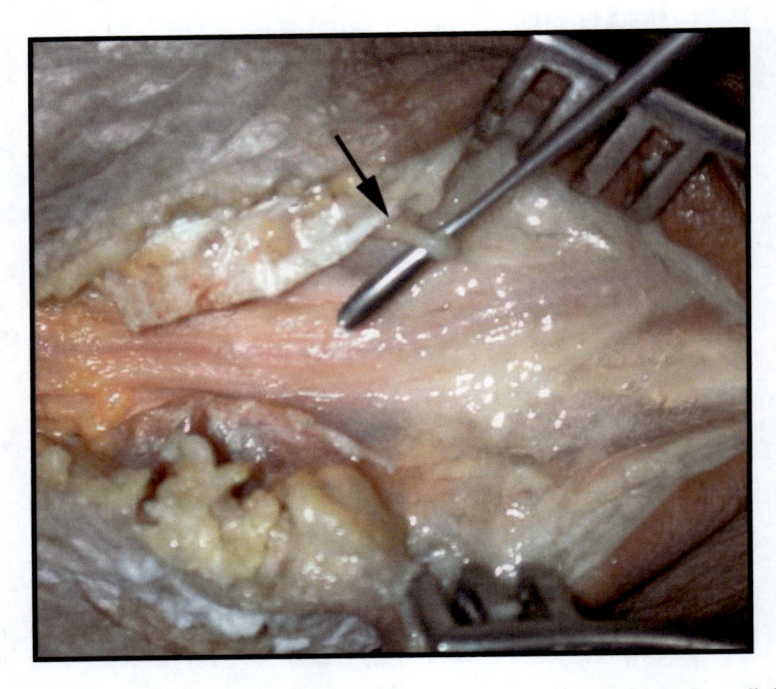

Figure 3. The median palmar cutaneous nerve (black arrow) arises from the radial side of the median nerve.

As the flexor muscles contract to bend the fingers downward into flexion towards the palm of the hand, the flexor tendons slide through the confined space within the carpal tunnel. The median palmar cutaneous nerve arises from the radial side of the median nerve approximately 5cm proximal to the TCL. This major sensory branch of the median nerve travels superficially to the carpal tunnel and provides major sensory innervation to the thenar eminence (Figure 3). The median nerve travels through the carpal tunnel alongside the flexor tendons and then divides into a motor branch that controls the thumb flexor and adductor muscles and sensory branches that provide over half the hand with the sensory of touch. The recurrent motor branch usually arises from the median nerve distal to the TCL, but anatomical variations have been reported. Three major variations are extraligamentous (50%), subligamentous (30%) and transligamentous (20%) based on their location compared to TCL [14, 15] (Figure 4).

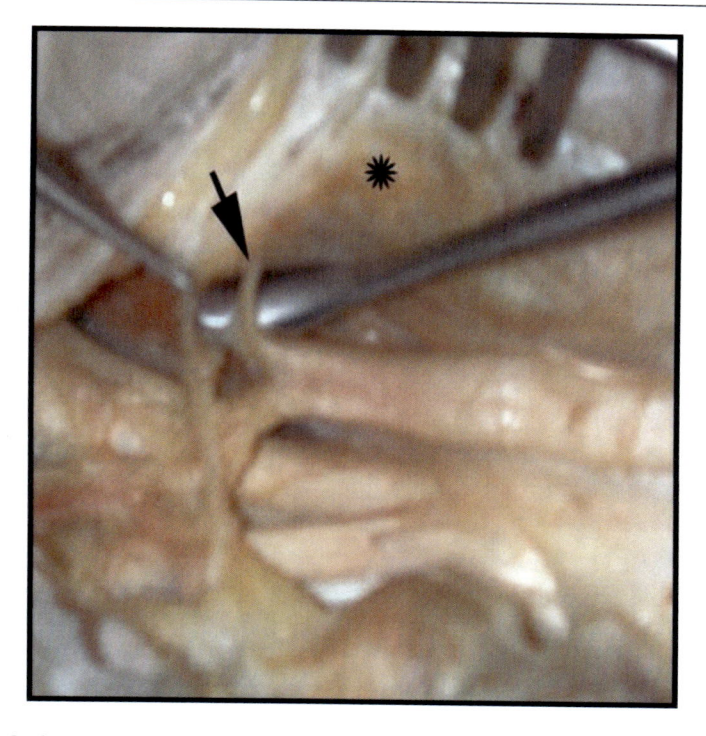

Figure 4. Cadaver dissection image shows the recurrent motor branch of the median nerve (black arrow) course through the transverse carpal ligament (asterisk).

Pathophysiology and Risk Factors Associated with CTS

Traditionally, idiopathic CTS has been reported to be caused by a mismatch between the size of the median nerve and the contents of the carpal tunnel, which leads to increased pressure within the carpal tunnel and disturbance in the blood flow to the median nerve. Compression of the nerve inside the carpal tunnel may induce venous congestion and subsequent edema; and prolonged epineurial edema causes fibroblast invasion into the affected tissue and subsequent formation of constricting scar tissue around the median nerve.

The nerve proximal to the compression site becomes enlarged because of an increase in the amount of endoneurial connective tissue, edema in the epineurium and endoneurial space, or obstruction of axoplasmic flow [16].

Mechanical Factors

Biomechanical studies show persistent nerve conduction impairment is due to the effects of nerve compression [17]. A "tadpole" lesion, characterized by thinning of the myelin, develops because of a shearing-type of pressure phenomenon at the end of the internodal segment with a bulbous-like swelling at the facing edge.

The carpal tunnel is dorsally and radio-ulnarly surrounded by the carpal bones and volarly surrounded by the TCL, through which run eight finger flexor tendons, the flexor pollicis longus tendon, the synovium, and the median nerve. The tendons transmit force generated by the forearm muscles to the digital phalanxes. These tendons pass through a flexor pulley system that includes the TCL and digital pulleys, where synovial fluid keeps friction between the tendon and pulleys low through both boundary and fluid film lubrication [18, 19].

In vivo measurements have revealed the tendon excursion to be 24–50 mm during active flexion and extension of the wrist and fingers. The excursion of the median nerve has also been measured: it has been found to range from 3 to 12 mm in preserved cadavers, from 9 to 14 mm in fresh frozen cadavers [20, 21], and from 11.0 to 28.8 mm during wrist and elbow movement in vivo [22].

In addition, the flexor tendons and median nerve move independently as well as concurrently in all anatomical directions (proximal-distal, radial-ulnar, and volar-dorsal directions). Different degrees of excursion between the flexor tendons and the median nerve could result in strain and micro-damage to the synovial tissue as well as the median nerve [23, 24]. Furthermore, shear modulus of the subsynovial connective tissue in CTS patients is found to be significantly higher than that in control subjects. This finding may be consistent with the fact that fibrosis of the synovial tissue within the carpal tunnel is often observed in CTS patients.

In one study, the tendon force was measured in vivo using a buckle-type transducer positioned over the carpal tunnel during pinching activities involving the thumb and digits; the maximum force recorded was 12.0 kgf, with a mean applied pinch force of 3.5 kgf. During active flexion of the digits, the flexor digitorum profundus and flexor pollicis longus tendons bear forces of 6.4 and 4.2 kgf, respectively [25]. Similar measurements were conducted in more recent studies, and similar values were reported. Because these values were measured after division of the TCL, the tendon force proximal to the TCL may have been even greater than that due to friction between the tendon and the TCL, which has been estimated to be around 0.1 N when an external force of 2 N is applied [26]. Furthermore, it is known that the flexor tendons move upward from the floor of the carpal tunnel during active finger movement [27-29]. This movement of the flexor tendons generates a compression (or reaction) force between the tendons and the TCL. On the basis of a theoretical model, it has been estimated that almost the same amount of force of the flexor tendon can be applied to the TCL during finger movement [30]. Those findings support the possibility of wear and degeneration of the tendon and the surrounding synovium during everyday activities, which are believed to play an important role in the development of idiopathic CTS; however, it remains unclear as to how much force or friction and how many cycles are needed to cause degeneration of the synovial tissue and flexor tendons and to affect the median nerve. Damage of the synovial tissue can be caused by factors such as the applied force and the duration and rate of loading, which are closely related to physical activity. Kursa et al. found that during high-precision, isometric pinch maneuvers with the fingers in a static condition the tendon forces are independent of the loading rate. This finding may facilitate the development of preventive strategies against tendinopathy of the flexor tendons and subsequent CTS.

Morphological Changes in Synovial Tissue

In many studies, microscopic histological examinations have been performed to examine alterations in the synovial tissue, including subsynovial connective tissue, around the flexor tendons. Only 10% of the synovial specimens resected from patients with idiopathic CTS exhibited inflammatory changes, but most exhibited edema or fibrosis [31]. Moreover, detailed histological examinations of synovial tissue obtained from CTS patients revealed an increase in fibroblast density, collagen fiber size, and vascular proliferation [32] and a decrease in the elastin content around the synovial vessels; these findings were indicative of chronic degeneration. Electron microscopic analyses of synovial tissue specimens obtained from patients with idiopathic CTS revealed deformed collagen fibrils with a spiral appearance, distinct from those in people without CTS; however, the process that leads to the altered morphology of the collagen fibrils remains to be clarified [33].

Biochemical Changes in Synovial Tissue

Mechanical stress applied to the synovial tissue inside the carpal tunnel can also cause biochemical alterations to the tissue. The expression of dermatan, keratan, and chondroitin sulfate in the synovium was compared between CTS patients and controls. Immunostaining revealed greater keratan reactivity in the tissues of CTS patients. This suggests that altered proteoglycan ratios may reduce the ability of the synovium to bear the compressive forces, thus increasing the force incident on the median nerve inside the carpal canal [34]. In addition, repetitive exposure of the tendons to compression or tensile strength can increase the proteoglycan content in the tendon matrix, thus causing metaplasia or hypertrophy of the tendon, which can in turn increase the pressure within the carpal tunnel [35].

In an attempt to elucidate the role of tenascin-C, which is often involved in tissue remodeling and vascular stenosis, in the pathogenesis of CTS, Tsujii et al. found that mechanical strain on the flexor tenosynovium regulates the production of tenascin-C by the synovial lining and connective tissue [33]. On the basis of these biomechanical and histological findings, it has been speculated that insult to the synovium and the flexor tendons due to aging or repetitive and forceful movement of the wrist and fingers could lead to degeneration of the synovium and the tendons, leading to enlargement of the carpal tunnel from the inner side. Thus, the volume of the carpal tunnel contents increases, leading to median nerve compression and, eventually, idiopathic carpal tunnel syndrome.

Secondary CTS Including Space Occupying Lesion

Many other conditions apart from idiopathic CTS can increase the pressure within the carpal tunnel and cause median nerve compression inside the tunnel; these conditions include abnormalities of the flexor tendons, synovium or the structure inside the median nerve and space-occupying lesions [36]. In patients with symptoms of CTS, the underlying pathology should always be scrutinized. Specific diseases that affect the synovium and can cause secondary CTS include diabetes, rheumatoid arthritis, sarcoidosis, purulent tenosynovitis, tuberculosis, systemic lupus erythematosus, hypo- or hyperthyroidism, gout, and amyloidosis.

Neuropathic factors, such as diabetes, alcoholism, vitamin toxicity or deficiency, and exposure to toxins, can play a role in eliciting CTS symptoms.

This is because they affect the median nerve without increasing the interstitial pressure within the carpal tunnel. In fact, diabetic patients have higher tendency to develop CTS due to lower threshold for nerve damage [37]. An increase in the carpal tunnel pressure due to space occupying lesions such as those associated with wrist fracture and/or dislocation, lunatomalacia, ganglions, lipoma, or synovial cysts can also cause CTS [38].

Diabetes

The number of diabetic patients has been increasing. More attention should be paid to the possibility of CTS in diabetic patients because of its peculiar etiology and varied responses to treatment. The prevalence of CTS in diabetic patients is extremely high: It is estimated to occur in 14% patients without diabetic polyneuropathies and in up to 30% of those with diabetic polyneuropathies [39]. The degree to which median nerve function can be recovered after CTR is less among diabetic patients than among nondiabetic persons [40]. The less favorable outcome of CTR in diabetic patients may be attributed to the loss of normal regenerative ability in the peripheral nerve because of microangiopathy, macrophage dysfunction, abnormalities in the retrograde cell body reaction, Schwann cell dysfunction, or decreased expression of neurotrophic factors and their receptors [41]. It is undoubtedly mandatory that the blood glucose levels of patients be well controlled after surgery to ensure better recovery of nerve function. In CTS patients with diabetes, surgery should be indicated after due consideration to not only the severity of the symptoms but also the regenerative ability of the median nerve.

Amyloid Deposition

The amyloidoses are a heterogeneous group of disorders that may present with a diverse spectrum of clinical manifestations. The disorders are characterized by tissue deposition of insoluble, misassembled fibril proteins that ultimately lead to the disruption of normal tissue structure and function.

Although carpal tunnel syndrome is common in the general population and is a nonspecific manifestation of familial amyloid polyneuropathy (FAP), when it does occur in patients with FAP the lesions tend to be more severe than in patients with idiopathic carpal tunnel syndrome [42]. This is due to endoneurial amyloid deposits that accompany the nerve entrapment under the carpal tunnel ligament. Focal nerve lesions other than median neuropathy at the wrist are rare. Amyloidosis causes CTS because of amyloid deposition not only within the peripheral nerve but also in the synovium of the flexor tendons in the carpal tunnel. Microglobulin amyloid causes median nerve palsy in the carpal tunnel of patients undergoing long-term hemodialysis. CTS can also appear as an initial symptom in transthyretin (TTR) amyloidosis. In previous studies, 10%–20% of all synovial biopsy specimens obtained from patients who underwent CTR exhibited amyloid deposition, and 59% of all the specimens with amyloid deposits tested positive for TTR amyloid [43, 44]. However, it could not be determined whether such TTR amyloid deposition was sufficient to cause CTS. In cases where amyloid deposits are identified in the tenosynovium during CTR, systemic amyloidosis rarely develops during long-term follow-up, although some patients definitely need special care to prevent systemic amyloidosis [45-47]. The term "idiopathic CTS" may not be appropriate if amyloidosis is identified as the cause of the CTS condition. Because TTR deposition on the synovium is more common in older patients, the possibility of such deposition being the primary cause of CTS cannot be ruled out. In such cases, further studies are needed to clarify whether any of the clinical, electrophysiological or imaging findings correspond to those of idiopathic CTS.

Pregnancy

Pregnancy and labor may lead to the development of peripheral nerve disorder, including CTS, facial nerve palsy, lumbosacral radiculopathy, meralgia paresthetica, and femoral neuropathy, among which CTS is the most frequently observed [48]. CTS may be caused by edema associated with fluid retention in the synovium, which exerts pressure on the median nerve. The true cause of pregnancy-related CTS is unknown. It is thought to be multifactorial, with median nerve compression resulting as a consequence of normal physiologic changes of pregnancy. Increased fluid volume, uterine pressure on the inferior vena cava, progesterone-mediated hyperemia, and fluid retention lead to generalized edema during pregnancy [49, 50]. Swelling in the carpal tunnel can cause compression of the median nerve. Specifically, pregnant patients with hand swelling that prevents them from wearing their rings have an increased incidence of carpal tunnel symptoms. In addition, patients who have gestational hypertension and preeclampsia have a higher incidence of CTS. Although there is a strong correlation of generalized increased volume load (generalized edema) and development of CTS, there is little evidence to support a direct correlation between weight gain during pregnancy and CTS. It has also been shown that patients nursing their infants postpartum have increased development of CTS [48].

Trigger Digit and CTS

Idiopathic CTS often accompanies tendon and synovial abnormalities at other sites. Trigger digit accompanies idiopathic CTS in approximately 20% of patients [51, 52]. If the primary lesion in idiopathic CTS is a synovial abnormality, as described above, it may lead to flexor tendon entrapment at the A1 pulley owing to enlargement of the tendon and its synovium. A recent prospective study has revealed a high prevalence of CTS in patients with trigger digit, wherein 91 of 211 patients with trigger digit (43%) had CTS [53]. Trigger digit occasionally develops after CTR with division of the TCL. This may be because of an alteration in the tendon mechanics, wherein the flexor tendon shifts volarly and increases the friction between the A1 pulley and the tendon. Although this hypothesis is probably accurate, further studies are required to prove it.

Clinical Symptom and Sign

Primary features of CTS include pain in the hand, unpleasant tingling, pain or numbness in the distal distribution of the median nerve (thumb, index, middle finger and the radial side of the ring finger), and a reduction of the grip strength and function of the affected hand. Symptoms tend to be worse at night, and clumsiness is reported during the day with activities requiring wrist flexion. Patients often describe a phenomenon termed the "flick sign", in which shaking or flicking their wrists relieves symptoms [54, 55].

Many patients report symptoms outside the distribution of the median nerve as well, which has been confirmed by a systematic study conducted by Stevens *et al.* In 159 hands of patients with electrodiagnostically confirmed CTS, symptoms were most commonly reported in both the median and ulnar digits more frequently than the median digits alone [56]. They also report location of symptoms in areas other than the digits. 21% of patients had forearm paraesthesias and pain; 13.8% reported elbow pain; 7.5% reported arm pain; 6.3% reported shoulder pain; and 0.6% reported neck pain.

Interestingly, trigger digit presentation accompanies idiopathic CTS in approximately 20% of patients.

A large multi-center study has confirmed that patients with mild to moderate CTS are more likely to report substantial symptoms and mild functional limitations, whereas patients with more severe disease may report less severe symptoms, but have more severe functional limitations of the hand [57]. This appears to be a contradiction, but in fact it relates to the fact that severe compromise of the median nerve may impair sensory functioning to the extent that the profound numbness minimizes the experience of tingling and pain. However, profound functional limitations will ensue as a result of numbness and motor impairment. Patients suffering from CTS often report subjective feelings of swelling in their hands or wrists, but no apparent swelling can be observed. However, some clinicians find that this symptom has some diagnostic value attached to it.

In study of over 8000 patients with suspected CTS, symptoms on the radial part of the hand and nocturnal exacerbation of symptoms were most strongly predictive of positive NCS [58, 59]. In a retrospective study of 1039 patients with a neurophysiological diagnosis of CTS, Nora et al., found that the most characteristic manifestation of the syndrome was parasthesia in the median nerve distribution, frequently extending to the whole hand. Pain was very common but less specific, and weakness was rare [60]. Phalen noted a volar wrist swelling in several patients – a visual and palpable swelling into the shape of a "hot dog". He studied this presentation in 82 hands with CTS and in 200 control hands, and found that it correlated well with Tinel and Phalen signs [61]. He concluded that it is a useful diagnostic sign, because it depends on clinical observation rather than the patient's history.

Some patients may present with atypical signs of CTS, such as "writer's cramp" or fatigue, pain in the shoulder only, cold sensitivity in the fingers (presumably reflecting the median nerve's supply of sympathetic fibers to part of the forearm and hand), forearm pain, or numbness in the third finger only. Sometimes there may be no symptoms but patients present with visual thenar atrophy (Figure 5) and denervation on nerve conduction studies.

In some instances, patients only have symptoms with rigorous activity, usually work-related, and present with minimal symptoms or objective findings when examined [62, 63].

This is termed "dynamic CTS" and patients usually benefit from conservative management, including alteration of work duties. Therefore, the importance of a well-defined history is particularly important in these cases.

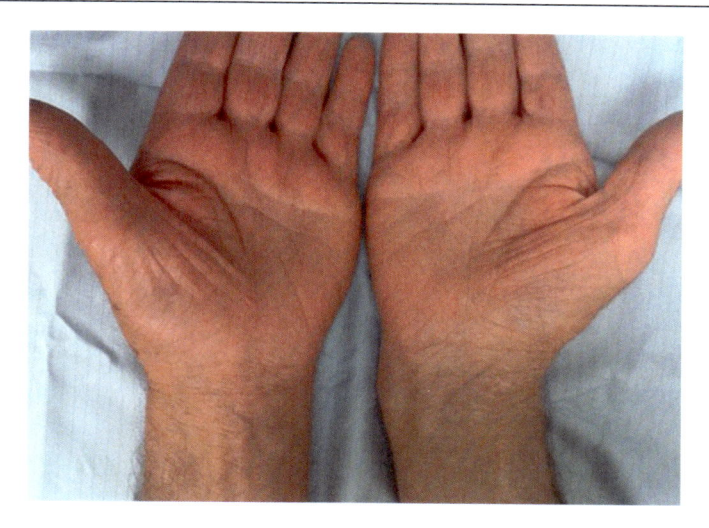

Figure 5. Clinical picture of the bilateral CTS patient shows thenar muscle atrophy on the left hand.

Diagnosis

Further testing is usually required to rule out other conditions that have similar symptoms. Further tests include:

Blood Tests

A blood test can determine if you have an underlying condition relating to CTS, such as diabetes, rheumatoid arthritis and underactive thyroid gland (hypothyroidism) [63].

Nerve Conduction Study

A nerve conduction study is a test that measures how fast signals are transmitted through nerves. During the test, electrodes (small metallic discs) are placed on the hand and wrist, which produce an electrical current that stimulates the nerves in the wrist, fingers and forearm. The results from the test will be used to assess any possible damage to the median nerve [64].

Electromyography

Electromyography (EMG) provides useful information about how well hand muscles are able to respond when a nerve is stimulated, indicating any nerve damage [65]. During the test, fine needles are inserted into the muscles. The needles detect any natural electrical activity given off by hand muscles. However, electromyography is rarely used for carpal tunnel syndrome in the UK because nerve conduction studies are usually able to confirm the diagnosis and measure the degree of damage to the nerve.

Electromyography and nerve conduction studies can help to establish how severely the median nerve is being compressed and the effect it is having on patient's symptoms.

Imaging Studies

An X-ray may be recommended, but usually only to aid in the diagnosis of fractures and other disorders such as rheumatoid arthritis. An X-ray is a procedure that produces images of the carpal bone and joint.

To thoroughly examine the structure of the median nerve inside of the carpal tunnel, ultrasound or MRI is recommended.

The use of ultrasound (US) has been implicated in the diagnosis of CTS because thickening of the median nerve, flattening of the nerve within the carpal tunnel and bowing of the flexor retinaculum are all features diagnostic of CTS [66].

Several studies have concluded that cross sectional area is the most predictive measurement, but there is some debate regarding the level within the tunnel that this measurement should be taken, and what constitutes abnormal values. The cross sectional area of the median nerve has been used in US to classify the severity of CTS as normal, mild, moderate and severe [67].

Magnetic resonance imaging (MRI) is excellent for picking up rare pathological causes of CTS such as ganglion, hemangioma or bony deformity – the presence of which may alter surgical strategy [68]. Furthermore, it is useful to understand the anatomic relationship of the neurovascular structures around the carpal tunnel, which is critical in preventing damage, thus leading to decreased morbidity [69, 70] (Figure 6).

MRI is able to predict those patients who would benefit from surgical intervention, because the length of the abnormal nerve signal on T2- weighted

MRI and the median-ulnar sensory latency difference are good predictors of surgical outcome. However, the results do not correlate well with patients' perceived severity of symptoms, mainly because MRI provides only anatomical information as opposed to information on nerve impairment and function [71].

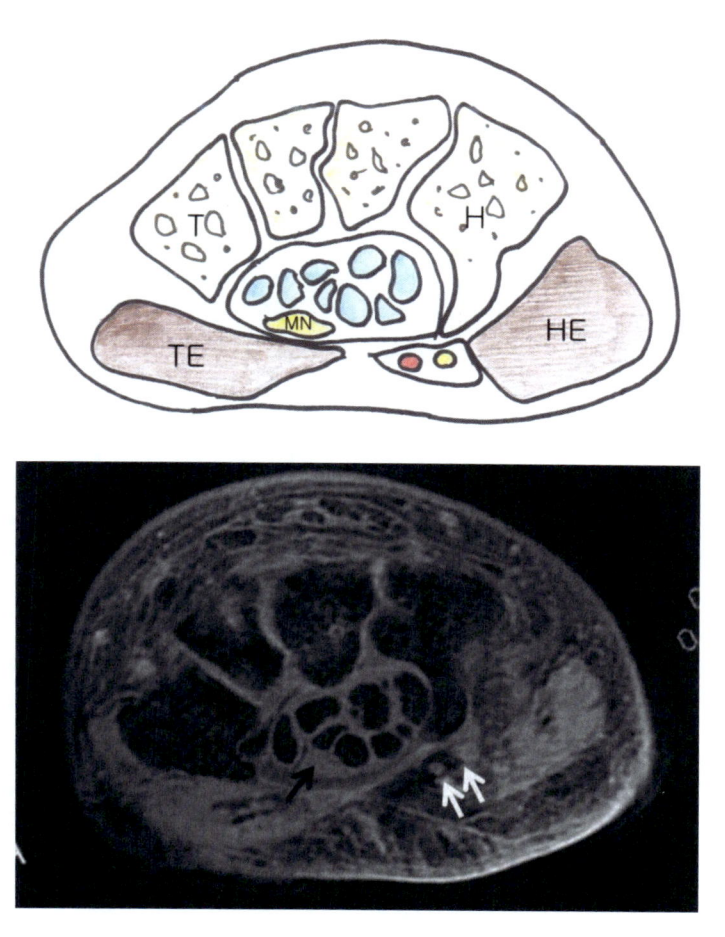

Figure 6. A) Schematic drawing of carpal tunnel shows the median nerve, flexor tendons and ulnar neurovascular structures around the carpal tunnel. T; trapezium, H; hamate, TE; thenar eminence, HE; hypothenar eminence, MN; median nerve B) MR imaging displays anatomy of the carpal tunnel on axial images, showing increased signal intensity of the median nerve (Black arrow) on T2-weighted images. Furthermore, it shows the anatomic relationship of the ulnar neurovascular structures (White arrows) around the carpal tunnel, which is critical in preventing damage during the surgical treatment.

Disadvantage of MRI is the cost of the study, and is therefore not routinely used. It is commonly used in determining the point of nerve entrapment after failure of initial carpal tunnel release, for differential diagnosis in the cases of ambiguous symptoms and to confirm the presence of space-occupying lesions.

Dynamic MRI study gives special interest to understand the location dynamics of neurovascular structures during the wrist motion. In the recent radiological study using dynamic MRI, there was substantial overlap of the contents of Guyon's canal across the transverse carpal ligament in a high proportion of patients [70]. With ulnar flexion of the wrist, there is a further radial displacement of these ulnar neurovascular structures, which may be more vulnerable to be injured in both open and endoscopic surgery (Figure 7).

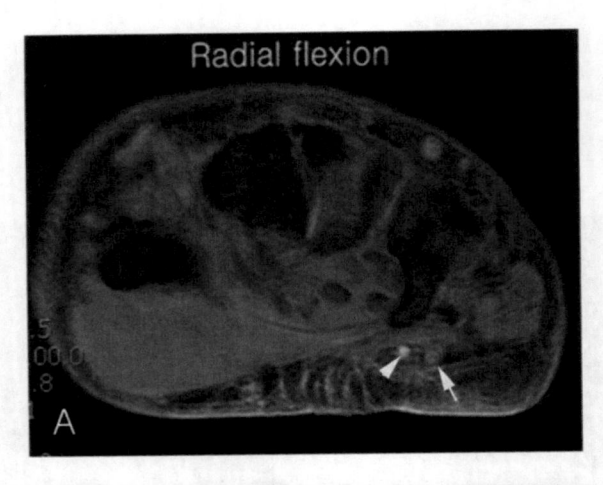

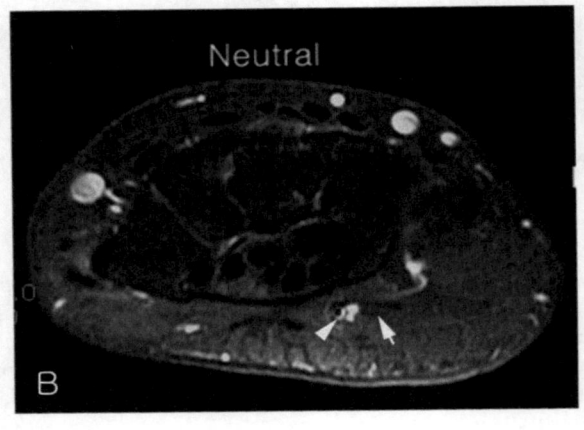

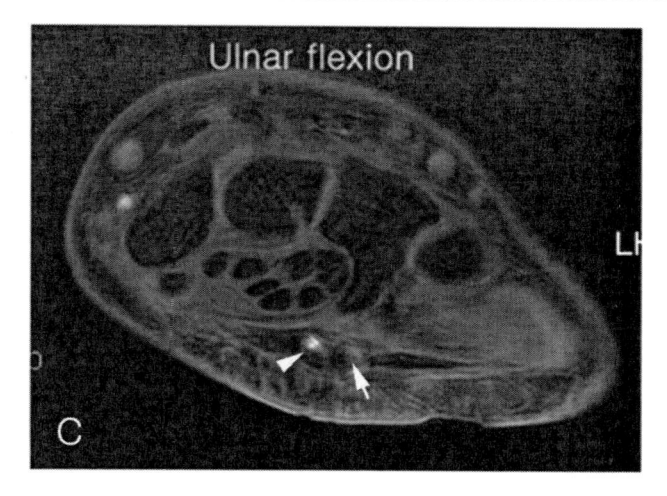

Figure 7. Magnetic resonance imaging with different wrist position reveals a dynamic displacement of the contents of Guyon's canal with changing wrist positions and a progressive radial migration of the ulnar neurosvascular structures as the wrist position moved from radial flexion (A) through neutral (B), and then to ulnar flexion (C) (arrowhead : ulnar artery, arrow : ulnar artery).

These anatomical relationships are important for endoscopic carpal tunnel surgery because the wrist position can change unintentionally during surgery when using local anesthesia. Therefore, this information about the dynamic changes in the location of the neurovascular structures will help to ensure optimal placement of the incision site for endoscopy and mini-open surgery, as well as to facilitate the least intrusive positioning of the endoscope.

Differential Diagnosis

While CTS is certainly the most common of the neuropathies to occur in the upper extremity, it is important to note other common compression neuropathies that can at times mimic CTS.

Cervical Radiculopathy

Cervical radiculopathy caused by cervical spondylosis most commonly occurs in middle-aged or elderly patients and C6 is the root with the greatest degree of nearly identical symptoms to those of median nerve compression

[72]. Common symptoms associated with cervical radiculopathy, that do not occur in CTS include: Neck and shoulder pain, especially when they occur with concurrent coughing or sneezing. Similarly, back pain, located at the medial border of the scapula is characteristic of a radiculopathy, and is not expected in CTS. Night pain, a common complaint of a patient with CTS, does not occur with a patient suffering from radiculopathy, daytime pain with arm use is the usual complaint. If the sixth cervical nerve is affected, there may be weakness of elbow flexion and wrist extension, the biceps reflex may be lost or reduced, and electromyographic (EMG) studies will show denervation out of median nerve territory if the cause of the disorder is cervical nerve root damage. Finally, utilizing the Semmes-Weinstein sensory test, the clinician would note a sensory loss of the C6 dermatome (thumb and lateral boarder of the upper extremity running to the neck), rather than the expected loss at the thumb, index, middle and radial half of the 4th digit. For further information regarding C6 radiculopathy, please refer to the radiculopathy standard of care.

Pronator Syndrome

Also a syndrome resulting from a compression of the medial nerve, the differences in symptoms are due in part to the site of compression [73]. In pronator syndrome, the medial nerve becomes compressed as it passes by the pronator muscle and the insertion of the deep flexor muscles at the elbow joint. With this syndrome, sensory loss will mimic that of CTS. However, there are several differences between the two diagnoses. The pronator syndrome is distinguished by exacerbation attributable to resisted pronation and passive supination activities, positive Tinel's sign at the proximal forearm overlying the median nerve, tenderness and paresthesias in the median nerve distribution on direct compression over pronator muscle, and pain and median nerve paresthesias with forced pronation, as well as passive supination at the limit of full elbow extension. Symptoms brought on by wrist movements, a hallmark of CTS are not common with pronator syndrome [74].

Raynaud's Disease

The symptoms caused by local vasospasm are differentiated from CTS in the sense that Raynaud's phenomenon does not involve any distinction between the fingers, with all the fingers and palm being equally affected.

Diminished circulation symptoms such as color blanching at the digits, and cool to the touch temperature of the hand can be observed on a patient with Raynaud's, while they are not observed in patients with CTS [75].

Cubital Tunnel Syndrome

Cubital tunnel syndrome is an ulnar nerve compression neuropathy resulting from acute or chronic external pressure on the ulnar nerve as it passes through the cubital tunnel during its course from the arm to the forearm [76, 77]. The cubital tunnel is formed by the condylar groove between the medial epicondyle of the humerus and the olecranon of the ulna. The symptoms of ulnar nerve compression will be quite different from ones caused by median nerve compression. Patients will usually describe a sharp or aching pain on the medial side the elbow, hand pain is not as common as it is in CTS. Sensory loss will be felt at the ring and small fingers, motor loss will be seen by atrophy of the 3rd and 4th lumbrical muscles. A more recognizable clinical feature is atrophy of the intrinsic muscles with clawing of the ring and little fingers.

Treatment

Conservative Treatment

Conservative treatment measures are unlikely to cure the condition of CTS but may alleviate the symptoms enough to obviate the need for surgical treatment.

Medical Treatment

Oral administration of NSAIDs and steroid can be used to reduce the synovial inflammation but their long-term medication needs to be evaluated in a risk-benefit manner for each patient [78]. The main side effect of corticosteroid is that it limits reduces collagen and proteoglycan synthesis, thus limiting tenocytes and hereby reducing the mechanical strength of the tendon, this leads to further degeneration. Pyridoxine or vitamin B6 has been used as a therapeutic agent. However, it has tended to be temporary.

Splint

Splinting of the wrist in the neutral position to 15 degree of extension is the initial intervention in the conservative treatment of CTS. Splinting the wrist in this position places the carpal tunnel in its most open position and allows for restoration of maximal circulation to the median nerve [79]. Further compression to the median nerve with prolonged wrist flexion while sleeping, or during daily/occupational activities are prevented with the use of a wrist splint. Based on what is known to date, current treatment for patients with mild to moderate CTS recommend including a conservative program of splinting the wrist in neutral for nocturnal wear. Typically pre-fabricated Velcro closed wrist splints are used. The occupational or physical therapist for the patient that is receiving therapy services typically fits this.

The wearing schedule of the splint is primarily recommended for nighttime use. Patients who are having complaints of constant symptoms, or who have pain and or sensory changes with activity are instructed to wear the splint at work or during highly resistive and repetitive motions. The patient is generally instructed to continue with the splint-wearing schedule for 4 to 6 weeks, and then gradually decrease splint use over the subsequent 4 weeks. Workers identified with CTS symptom surveillance tended to benefit from a 6-week nocturnal splinting trial, and the benefits were still evident at the 1-year follow up. Length of time for splint use may also be determined by the causes of the individual's CTS's and their response to treatment. For example, a patient demonstrating CTS symptoms during pregnancy may only require splinting during this time. Long-term use of a splint (longer than 2 months) may be indicated when other conservative measures have been exhausted, and the patient declines surgical or other medical intervention.

If a patient is unable to comfortably fit into a pre- fabricated splint, or if the correct wrist position cannot be achieved due to wrist deformity, or unusual wrist size, a custom orthoplast splint may be fabricated. Either an occupational therapist or physical therapist fabricates this custom splint for the patient. As with the pre-fabricated splint, the wrist should be placed in the neutral to 15 degrees of extension position. If a patient's symptoms do not positively respond to basic custom wrist splinting, recent studies have shown a benefit to extending the orthoplast splint distally to include the patient's metacarpophalangeal joints (MCP's) in extension. This splint immobilizes the MCP's and does not allow for the lumbrical muscles (intrinsic hand muscles responsible for MCP flexion) to rest within the tunnel. The splint-wearing schedule for this splint would mimic the schedule for the wrist splint, however, the patient should be instructed to remove this splint periodically throughout the day for mobilization of the MCP's, and tendon gliding exercises (see below) to eliminate the possibility of creating joint stiffness.

Injection Treatment

The injection of steroid preparations into the carpal canal is a recognized practice in the management of carpal tunnel syndrome. Local corticosteroid injection for carpal tunnel syndrome provides greater clinical improvement in symptoms one month after injection compared to placebo [80]. However, significant symptom relief beyond one month has not been demonstrated in the literature.

And also, this procedure could be associated with a risk of temporary or permanent damage to the median nerve. Therefore, its role should be limited to a diagnostic aid in cases in which symptoms are atypical, a temporizing agent in patients with severe symptoms either who are awaiting surgery or in whom spontaneous remission might be expected, and as a definitive treatment in patients who do not desire surgery. Injection should be performed using proper technique by physicians skilled in carpal tunnel surgery. A soluble preparation of dexamethasone is recommended. Immediate paresthesia in the median nerve distribution or exacerbation of symptoms beyond 48 hours following injection is suspect for inadvertent nerve injury; therefore, early surgical decompression is indicated.

Surgical Treatment

There have been several different approaches to decompressing the carpal tunnel over the years, from OCTR, to more limited-open approaches using commercially available products, to endoscopic techniques [81-83].

Regardless of the surgical technique selected, all structures to be incised should be seen and identified during the procedure. Furthermore, the safety of the median nerve needs to be verified before any type of carpal tunnel release.

Open Carpal Tunnel Release

The incision used for the open carpal tunnel release should be in a proper position to reach the transverse ligament easily. At the same time, vigilance is required and abnormal anatomy should always be considered. The incision should be at safe distance from the recurrent motor branch of median nerve, major sensory branches of the median and ulnar nerves (palmar cutaneous branch of the median and ulnar nerve), superficial palmar arch (Figure 8), ulnar artery and nerve, which could be vulnerable to be damaged. In other words, determination of the incision location is of critical importance in the carpal tunnel surgery.

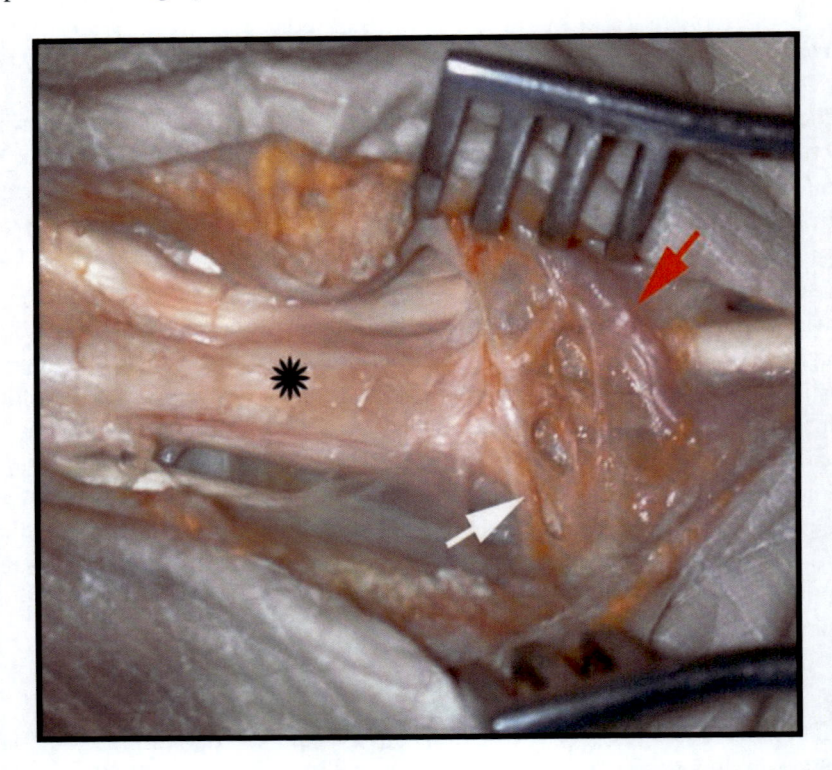

Figure 8. Cadaver picture demonstrates the median nerve (asterisk) after the resection of the transverse carpal ligament (TCL). The location of the superficial palar arch (Black arrows) is just distal to the TCL (C). P; proximal, D; distal, R; radial, U; ulnar.

The thenar creases takes variable course, palmar incision should be located ulnar side to thenar crease to avoid the palmar cutaneous branch of median nerve, because this branch always originated medial side of the median nerve and course along the medial margin.

Curvilinear incision of traditional open carpal tunnel release is not recommended nowadays because the palmar cutaneous branch of median nerve may be more risky proximally and some wound-related symptoms may persist (Figure 9A).

As for mini-open carpal tunnel release, a 1.5 cm longitudinal incision was placed 0.5 cm proximal to a transverse line from the ulnar side of the abducted thumb, bisecting the axis of the ring finger, or ulnar to thenar crease (Figure

9B). The palmar fascia was divided in line with the skin incision. The deep transverse carpal ligament (TCL) was identified, and incised with blade as a small hole.

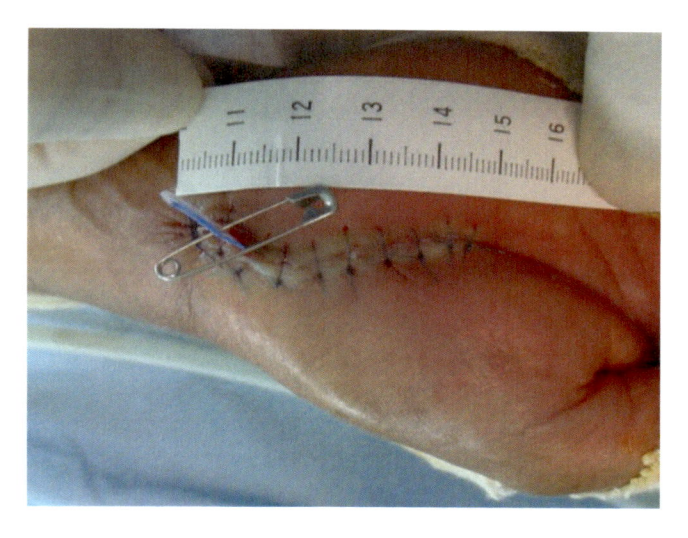

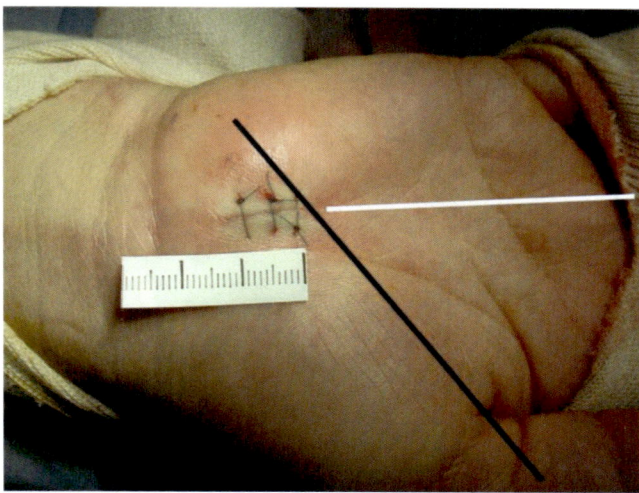

Figure 9. (A) The traditional open carpal tunnel release (OCTR) procedure consists of a long, palmar curvilinear incision to divide the transverse carpal ligament. (B) Mini-open carpal tunnel release. Proposed incision measuring 1.5cm starts and extends distally at the intersection of Kaplan's cardinal line (black line) and a line drawn along the radial border of the ring finger (white line).

After that, a small blunt tip clamp was passed through this hole from proximal to distal direction for protection of underlying median nerve. A blade was placed over the clamp and used to release distal edge of TCL under direct vision to avoid injury to thenar branch of the median nerve and the vascular arch. It is important to be aware of potential anomalies: connection between the flexor pollicis longus and the index flexor digitorum profundus tendon, interconnection between the median nerve and the ulnar nerve. Wherever proximal edge was divided by blunt tip scissors, a blind technique from ulnar to Palmaris longus to avoid injury to palmar cutaneous branch of median nerve was used. The skin was closed with 5-0 Nylon using about three stitches and a compression dressing was applied. Then, the tourniquet was released.

Endoscopic Carpal Tunnel Release

For the past decade, the only therapy for this condition was the conventional open carpal tunnel release (OCTR) procedure. However, since several investigators reported success with endoscopic decompression in the late 1980s, ECTR has gained rapid popularity as a substitute therapy for CTS [83-85].

The often cited advantages of endoscopic decompression are the reduction of post-surgical pain at the incision site, superior aesthetic results due to a smaller surgical scar, and the rapid recovery of muscle power of the carpal joint resulting in reduced associated costs [86]. However, according to numerous investigators, endoscopic decompression is not without risks. Complications such as the erroneous insertion of the endoscope into Guyon's canal oftentimes results in injury to the ulnar nerve and/or nearby blood vessels, and the insufficient incision of TCL [87, 88].

Although the frequency of complications varies according to the study, it has been reported that the difference in outcomes of endoscopic surgery is closely associated with the experience level as well as the anatomical knowledge of the surgeon [89].

Therefore, successful minimally invasive carpal tunnel decompression therapy including endoscopic surgery requires the surgeon not only to be adept with the surgical instrumentation but also to possess a thorough anatomical understanding by performing autopsies [90, 91]. The structures that are generally known to be readily injured during endoscopic surgery for CTS are the ulnar nerve and blood vessels in Guyon's canal, the palmar cutaneous branch of the median nerve, the recurrent motor branch of the median nerve, the superficial palmar communication between the median and ulnar nerves so called Berrettini branch, and the superficial palmar arch between the radial and ulnar arteries [91, 92].

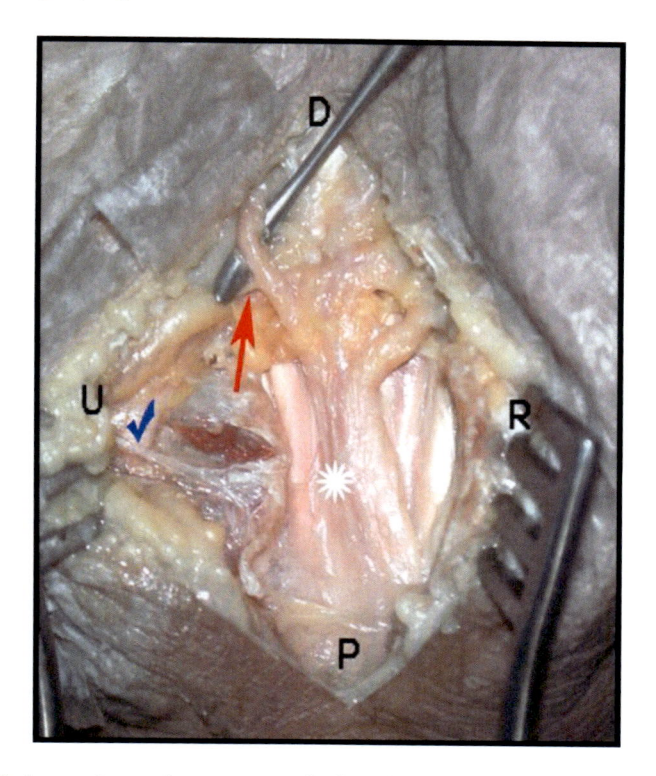

Figure 10. Cadaver picture demonstrates the location of the Berretini's branch (arrow). Superficial palmar communication, also known as the Berrettini branch is communicating nerve branch between the median (asterisk) and ulnar nerves (check mark). P; proximal, D; distal, R; radial, U; ulnar.

Among the structures described above, the superficial palmar arch, the palmar cutaneous branch of the median nerve, and the ulnar nerve within Guyon's canal were located over 5 mm apart from the penetration route of endoscopy during carpal tunnel decompression and thus they were considered to be rather safe. However, as the Berrettini branch is located in close proximity to the distal margin of the TCL (Figure 10) and as there exists variation of the ulnar artery which deviates from Guyon's canal to the carpal tunnel, these structures may be directly in the path of the endoscope. Also, origins of the recurrent motor branch may locate proximal to the distal TCL in some cases. If the endoscopic device is levered away from the ring finger to gain access radially (using the index or long finger access approach), such a movement could possibly endanger the recurrent motor branch. Therefore, the recurrent motor branch of the median nerve, the Berrettini branch, and the radially-deviated ulnar artery are considered to be the most vulnerable structures in endoscopic decompression.

The recurrent motor branch of the median nerve has an extraligamentous course in 46% of cases, travels subligamentously in 31% of cases, and travels transligamentously in 23% cases [93]. The latter two variants are at risk for being damaged during ECTR. However, most recurrent motor branches originate from the superolateral portion of the median nerve. So, if the passage of the endoscopy material is along the ulnar side of the median nerve during ECTR, injuries to the recurrent motor branch can be avoided.

To date, in association with endoscopic decompression, reports on the anatomical variations of nerve structures in the vicinity of carpal tunnel are abundant. However, information pertinent to the vascular structures is relatively rare in that area [94]. To determine how significant a problem vascular damage is in ECTR, Palmer reviewed complications of endoscopic and open carpal tunnel release over a 5-year period in the United States of America, and found that in contrast to OCTR, the most frequent complication from performing the endoscopic carpal tunnel release procedure was vessel laceration [88]. It is clearly understood that Guyon's canal (with the enclosed ulnar nerve and artery) lies radial to the pisiform and therefore directly superficial to the carpal tunnel in its proximal portion. Distally, however, the canal has been described as taking a curved course, with the ulnar nerve and artery traveling ulnar to the hook of the hamate [70, 91]. Several radiologic studies using computed tomography (CT) and magnetic resonance imaging (MRI) have accurately described some of the anatomy of the carpal tunnel and its relation to Guyon's canal [70, 95]. On perusal of the various radiographic scans in these articles, it became apparent to us that the distal portion of Guyon's canal held a variable relationship with the deeper structures, namely the hook of the hamate and the carpal tunnel. In the distal portion of the canal, splayed and branched neurovascular structures might perhaps be more vulnerable to injury by both the open technique of carpal tunnel release and the endoscopist's blade working from deep within the carpal tunnel. In one cadaveric study, the ulnar artery with radial deviation from Guyon's canal toward the carpal tunnel was detected in 29% (11/38) of the hands studied. In the 11 hands with this the deviation, the ulnar artery deviated by a maximum of 4 mm while in the neutral position. In comparison, in relation to the lateral margin of the hamate, and during ulnar flexion of wrist, the ulnar artery deviated by a maximum of 7 mm towards the carpal tunnel, while during radial flexion, the deviation towards the inside of the carpal tunnel decreased [91].

Considering the stiffness of cadavers, they concluded that in actual living patients, the difference may be significantly greater during ulnar and radial flexion, and thus it may be safer to transect the ligament with the wrist in radial flexion during TCL resection, and to avoid sectioning the TCL under the condition of ulnar flexion. One cadaveric study recommended that one should incise an area over 4 mm apart from the lateral margin of the hamate hook to avoid injuring of blood vessels due to anatomical variations of the ulnar artery may be that during the resection of the TCL. The ulnar artery is more prone to be caught as the scalpel is withdrawn when the wrist is placed in ulnar flexion and when placing the edge of the blade toward the ulnar side during ECTR. The endoscopy insertion area should be as far away from Guyon's canal as possible by placing the skin incision area of the upper part of the carpal tunnel just to the medial side of the radially-retracted Palmaris longus tendon.

Recurrent Carpal Tunnel Syndrome

The incidence of recurrent or persistent carpal tunnel syndrome is rare, although likely underestimated. Complications and failures are reported to occur in 3% to 25% of cases. Typically, complications of CTR can arise because of iatrogenic injuries to nerves (palmar cutaneous branch of median nerve, median nerve and ulnar nerve), vessels, or tendons (including adhesions to the adjacent tissues) as well as bowstringing of the flexor tendon. Pillar pain and complex regional pain syndrome are complications that are not completely understood. Infection, hematoma, skin necrosis, and scar hypertrophy are other additionally reported complications of CTR [96].

Persistent symptoms were often related to incomplete release of the transverse carpal ligament, especially with endoscopic techniques. Although incomplete release was the most common cause, other causes of persistent symptom after CTR included tenosynovitis and fibrosis at the surgical site [97].

An incorrect primary diagnosis can also be a cause for an apparent postoperative persistence of CTS. Conditions like cervical radiculopathy; spinal cord lesions; proximal nerve compressive lesions, such as pronator syndrome, thoracic outlet syndrome, brachial plexus lesions; or systemic disease, such as diabetes, hypothyroidism, and hemodialysis-related neurologic sequelae, may manifest with symptoms similar to that of CTS [98].

Complaints of worsening numbness, tingling, or weakness should alert the physician to possible nerve injury and need for early exploration. The overall results of revision carpal tunnel procedures are less successful than primary surgery; however, surgery should be performed when indicated, as it may alleviate or improve symptoms.

In most cases of recurrent or persistent carpal tunnel syndrome, conservative treatments will not provide adequate relief. Therefore strong consideration should be given to evaluate the exact cause of failure and re-explore the carpal tunnel. For the treatment of failed carpal tunnel release, it is essential to make the correct diagnosis of recurrent or persistent CTS.

The revision carpal tunnel surgery begins by extending the previous incision into normal tissue to allow proximal and distal identification of the median nerve to first facilitate exploration. Following release of the ligament and neurolysis, a decision must be made whether to provide coverage in attempt to promote glide and minimize recurrent scar formation [99]. The decision is often dependent on the nerve mobility, position, and local soft tissue. If incomplete release of the ligament is felt to be the cause of the patient's symptoms, then no further treatment is needed and outcomes are expected to be similar to primary carpal tunnel release.

References

[1]   Gerritsen AA, Uitdehaag BM, van Geldere D, Scholten RJ, de Vet HC, Bouter LM. Systematic review of randomized clinical trials of surgical treatment for carpal tunnel syndrome. *The British journal of surgery.* 2001;88(10):1285-95.

[2]   Higgins JP, Graham TJ. Carpal tunnel release via limited palmar incision. *Hand clinics.* 2002;18(2):299-306.

[3]   Doyle JR, Carroll RE. The carpal tunnel syndrome. A review of 100 patients treated surgically. *California medicine.* 1968;108(4):263-7.

[4]   Spinner M, Spencer PS. Nerve compression lesions of the upper extremity. A clinical and experimental review. *Clinical orthopaedics and related research.* 1974(104):46-67.

[5]   Eason SY, Belsole RJ, Greene TL. Carpal tunnel release: analysis of suboptimal results. *Journal of hand surgery.* 1985;10(3):365-9.

[6]   Gelberman RH, Rydevik BL, Pess GM, Szabo RM, Lundborg G. Carpal tunnel syndrome. A scientific basis for clinical care. *The Orthopedic clinics of North America.* 1988;19(1):115-24.

[7]   Entin MA. Carpal tunnel syndrome and its variants. *The Surgical clinics of North America.* 1968;48(5):1097-112.

[8]   Willis CB, Alderman A, Louis DS. Anatomic anomalies and carpal tunnel syndrome: a review. *Techniques in hand & upper extremity surgery.* 1999;3(2):99-104.

[9]   Mackinnon SE, Dellon AL. Anatomic investigations of nerves at the wrist: I. Orientation of the motor fascicle of the median nerve in the carpal tunnel. *Annals of plastic surgery.* 1988;21(1):32-5.

[10]   Blair SJ. Avoiding complications of surgery for nerve compression syndromes. *The Orthopedic clinics of North America.* 1988;19(1):125-30.

[11]   Kretschmer T, Antoniadis G, Richter HP, Konig RW. Avoiding iatrogenic nerve injury in endoscopic carpal tunnel release. *Neurosurgery clinics of North America.* 2009;20(1):65-71, vi-vii.

[12]   Cooney WP. Tendon transfer for median nerve palsy. *Hand clinics.* 1988;4(2):155-65.

[13]   Thoma A, Veltri K, Haines T, Duku E. A systematic review of reviews comparing the effectiveness of endoscopic and open carpal tunnel decompression. *Plastic and reconstructive surgery.* 2004;113(4):1184-91.

[14]   Demircay E, Civelek E, Cansever T, Kabatas S, Yilmaz C. Anatomic variations of the median nerve in the carpal tunnel: a brief review of the literature. *Turkish neurosurgery.* 2011;21(3):388-96.

[15]   Rotman MB, Donovan JP. Practical anatomy of the carpal tunnel. *Hand clinics.* 2002;18(2):219-30.

[16]   Genba K, Ugawa Y, Kanazawa I, Okutsu I, Hamanaka I. Physiological assessment of endoscopic surgery for carpal tunnel syndrome. *Muscle & nerve.* 1993;16(5):567-8.

[17]   El-Karabaty H, Hetzel A, Galla TJ, Horch RE, Lucking CH, Glocker FX. The effect of carpal tunnel release on median nerve flattening and nerve conduction. *Electromyography and clinical neurophysiology.* 2005;45(4):223-7.

[18]   Uchiyama S, Itsubo T, Nakamura K, Kato H, Yasutomi T, Momose T. Current concepts of carpal tunnel syndrome: pathophysiology, treatment, and evaluation. *Journal of orthopaedic science : official journal of the Japanese Orthopaedic Association.* 2010;15(1):1-13.

[19] Uchiyama S, Yasutomi T, Fukuzawa T, Nakagawa H, Kamimura M, Kato H. Reducing neurologic and vascular complications of endoscopic carpal tunnel release using a modified chow technique. Arthroscopy : the journal of arthroscopic & related surgery : *official publication of the Arthroscopy Association of North America and the International Arthroscopy Association.* 2007;23(8):816-21.

[20] Coppieters MW, Alshami AM. Longitudinal excursion and strain in the median nerve during novel nerve gliding exercises for carpal tunnel syndrome. *Journal of orthopaedic research : official publication of the Orthopaedic Research Society.* 2007;25(7):972-80.

[21] Tuzuner S, Ozkaynak S, Acikbas C, Yildirim A. Median nerve excursion during endoscopic carpal tunnel release. *Neurosurgery.* 2004; 54(5):1155-60; discussion 60-1.

[22] Ugbolue UC, Nicol AC. A wrist tendon travel assessment of hand movements associated with industrial repetitive activities. *Work.* 2012;42(3):311-20.

[23] Henderson J, Thoreson A, Yoshii Y, Zhao KD, Amadio PC, An KN. Finite element model of subsynovial connective tissue deformation due to tendon excursion in the human carpal tunnel. *Journal of biomechanics.* 2011;44(1):150-5.

[24] Keir PJ, Bach JM. Flexor muscle incursion into the carpal tunnel: a mechanism for increased carpal tunnel pressure? *Clinical biomechanics.* 2000;15(5):301-5.

[25] Schuind F, Garcia-Elias M, Cooney WP, 3rd, An KN. Flexor tendon forces: in vivo measurements. *The Journal of hand surgery.* 1992;17(2):291-8.

[26] Zhao C, Ettema AM, Osamura N, Berglund LJ, An KN, Amadio PC. Gliding characteristics between flexor tendons and surrounding tissues in the carpal tunnel: a biomechanical cadaver study. *Journal of orthopaedic research : official publication of the Orthopaedic Research Society.* 2007;25(2):185-90.

[27] Kiritsis PG, Kline SC. Biomechanical changes after carpal tunnel release: a cadaveric model for comparing open, endoscopic, and step-cut lengthening techniques. *The Journal of hand surgery.* 1995;20(2):173-80.

[28] Netscher D, Dinh T, Cohen V, Thornby J. Division of the transverse carpal ligament and flexor tendon excursion: open and endoscopic carpal tunnel release. *Plastic and reconstructive surgery.* 1998;102(3):773-8.

[29] Brown RK, Peimer CA. Changes in digital flexor tendon mechanics after endoscopic and open carpal tunnel releases in cadaver wrists. *The Journal of hand surgery*. 2000;25(1):112-9.

[30] Uchiyama S, Amadio PC, Berglund LJ, An KN. Analysis of the gliding pattern of the canine flexor digitorum profundus tendon through the A2 pulley. *Journal of biomechanics*. 2008;41(6):1281-8.

[31] Nakamichi K, Tachibana S. Histology of the transverse carpal ligament and flexor tenosynovium in idiopathic carpal tunnel syndrome. The *Journal of hand surgery*. 1998;23(6):1015-24.

[32] Jinrok O, Zhao C, Amadio PC, An KN, Zobitz ME, Wold LE. Vascular pathologic changes in the flexor tenosynovium (subsynovial connective tissue) in idiopathic carpal tunnel syndrome. *Journal of orthopaedic research : official publication of the Orthopaedic Research Society*. 2004;22(6):1310-5.

[33] Tsujii M, Hirata H, Yoshida T, Imanaka-Yoshida K, Morita A, Uchida A. Involvement of tenascin-C and PG-M/versican in flexor tenosynovial pathology of idiopathic carpal tunnel syndrome. *Histology and histopathology*. 2006;21(5):511-8.

[34] Tucci M, Sud V, Freeland A. Compression of the median nerve in CTS is mediated by periods of acute synovial swelling. *Biomedical sciences instrumentation*. 2001;37:299-303.

[35] Yoon JH, Halper J. Tendon proteoglycans: biochemistry and function. *Journal of musculoskeletal & neuronal interactions*. 2005;5(1):22-34.

[36] Cobb TK, Cooney WP, An KN. Pressure dynamics of the carpal tunnel and flexor compartment of the forearm. *The Journal of hand surgery*. 1995;20(2):193-8.

[37] Lekholm C, Sundkvist G, Lundborg G, Dahlin L. [The diabetic hand-- complications of diabetes]. *Lakartidningen*. 2001;98(4):306-12.

[38] Sarawagi R, Anderson GA, Cherian RS. Fibrolipomatous hamartoma of the median nerve presenting with carpal tunnel syndrome. *Neurology India*. 2009;57(3):361-2.

[39] Perkins BA, Olaleye D, Bril V. Carpal tunnel syndrome in patients with diabetic polyneuropathy. *Diabetes care*. 2002;25(3):565-9.

[40] Ozkul Y, Sabuncu T, Kocabey Y, Nazligul Y. Outcomes of carpal tunnel release in diabetic and non-diabetic patients. *Acta neurologica Scandinavica*. 2002;106(3):168-72.

[41] Kennedy JM, Zochodne DW. Impaired peripheral nerve regeneration in diabetes mellitus. Journal of the peripheral nervous system : *JPNS*. 2005;10(2):144-57.

[42] Shin SC, Robinson-Papp J. Amyloid neuropathies. The Mount Sinai journal of medicine, New York. 2012;79(6):733-48.

[43] Stein K, Storkel S, Linke RP, Goebel HH. Chemical heterogeneity of amyloid in the carpal tunnel syndrome. Virchows Archiv A, *Pathological anatomy and histopathology*. 1987;412(1):37-45.

[44] Nakamichi KI, Tachibana S. Amyloid deposition in the synovium and ligament in idiopathic carpal tunnel syndrome. *Muscle & nerve*. 1996;19(10):1349-51.

[45] Murakami T, Tachibana S, Endo Y, Kawai R, Hara M, Tanase S, et al. Familial carpal tunnel syndrome due to amyloidogenic transthyretin His 114 variant. *Neurology*. 1994;44(2):315-8.

[46] Kyle RA, Gertz MA, Linke RP. Amyloid localized to tenosynovium at carpal tunnel release. Immunohistochemical identification of amyloid type. *American journal of clinical pathology*. 1992;97(2):250-3.

[47] Takei Y, Hattori T, Gono T, Tokuda T, Saitoh S, Hoshii Y, et al. Senile systemic amyloidosis presenting as bilateral carpal tunnel syndrome. Amyloid : *the international journal of experimental and clinical investigation : the official journal of the International Society of Amyloidosis*. 2002;9(4):252-5.

[48] Draper L. Pregnant women in the workplace: distinguishing between normal and abnormal physiologic changes. *AAOHN journal : official journal of the American Association of Occupational Health Nurses*. 2006;54(5):217-23; quiz 24-5.

[49] Seror P. Pregnancy-related carpal tunnel syndrome. *Journal of hand surgery*. 1998;23(1):98-101.

[50] al Qattan MM, Manktelow RT, Bowen CV. Pregnancy-induced carpal tunnel syndrome requiring surgical release longer than 2 years after delivery. *Obstetrics and gynecology*. 1994;84(2):249-51.

[51] Hombal JW, Owen R. Carpal tunnel decompression and trigger digits. *The Hand*. 1970;2(2):192-6.

[52] Hayashi M, Uchiyama S, Toriumi H, Nakagawa H, Kamimura M, Miyasaka T. Carpal tunnel syndrome and development of trigger digit. Journal of clinical neuroscience : *official journal of the Neurosurgical Society of Australasia*. 2005;12(1):39-41.

[53] Ryzewicz M, Wolf JM. Trigger digits: principles, management, and complications. *The Journal of hand surgery*. 2006;31(1):135-46.

[54] Todnem K, Lundemo GH. [Symptoms and clinical course in carpal tunnel syndrome]. *Tidsskrift for den Norske laegeforening : tidsskrift for praktisk medicin, ny raekke*. 2001;121(12):1489-92.

[55] Gupta SK, Benstead TJ. Symptoms experienced by patients with carpal tunnel syndrome. *The Canadian journal of neurological sciences Le journal canadien des sciences neurologiques.* 1997;24(4):338-42.

[56] Stevens JC. AAEM minimonograph #26: the electrodiagnosis of carpal tunnel syndrome. American Association of Electrodiagnostic Medicine. *Muscle & nerve.* 1997;20(12):1477-86.

[57] Katz JN, Fossel KK, Simmons BP, Swartz RA, Fossel AH, Koris MJ. Symptoms, functional status, and neuromuscular impairment following carpal tunnel release. *The Journal of hand surgery.* 1995;20(4):549-55.

[58] Kinura I, Kogure K. [Electrophysiological aspects of 639 symptomatic extremities with carpal tunnel syndrome]. *Rinsho shinkeigaku = Clinical neurology.* 1984;24(8):806-12.

[59] Mizumoto D, Hashizume H, Senda M, Nagoshi M, Inoue H. Electrophysiological assessment of the carpal tunnel syndrome in hemodialysis patients: formula for predicting surgical results. *Journal of orthopaedic science : official journal of the Japanese Orthopaedic Association.* 2003;8(1):8-15.

[60] Nora DB, Becker J, Ehlers JA, Gomes I. Clinical features of 1039 patients with neurophysiological diagnosis of carpal tunnel syndrome. *Clinical neurology and neurosurgery.* 2004;107(1):64-9.

[61] Phalen GS. Reflections on 21 years' experience with the carpal-tunnel syndrome. *JAMA : the journal of the American Medical Association.* 1970;212(8):1365-7.

[62] Goss BC, Agee JM. Dynamics of intracarpal tunnel pressure in patients with carpal tunnel syndrome. *The Journal of hand surgery.* 2010;35(2):197-206.

[63] Elliott B. Diagnosing and treating hypothyroidism. The Nurse practitioner. 2000;25(3):92-4, 9-105.

[64] Seror P. Nerve conduction studies after treatment for carpal tunnel syndrome. *Journal of hand surgery.* 1992;17(6):641-5.

[65] Ubogu EE, Benatar M. Electrodiagnostic criteria for carpal tunnel syndrome in axonal polyneuropathy. *Muscle & nerve.* 2006;33(6):747-52.

[66] Ajeena IM, Al-Saad RH, Al-Mudhafar A, Hadi NR, Al-Aridhy SH. Ultrasonic assessment of females with carpal tunnel syndrome proved by nerve conduction study. *Neural plasticity.* 2013;2013:754564.

[67] Chen SF, Lu CH, Huang CR, Chuang YC, Tsai NW, Chang CC, et al. Ultrasonographic median nerve cross-section areas measured by 8-point "inching test" for idiopathic carpal tunnel syndrome: a correlation of

nerve conduction study severity and duration of clinical symptoms. *BMC medical imaging.* 2011;11:22.

[68] Martins RS, Siqueira MG, Simplicio H, Agapito D, Medeiros M. Magnetic resonance imaging of idiopathic carpal tunnel syndrome: correlation with clinical findings and electrophysiological investigation. *Clinical neurology and neurosurgery.* 2008;110(1):38-45.

[69] Pasternack, II, Malmivaara A, Tervahartiala P, Forsberg H, Vehmas T. Magnetic resonance imaging findings in respect to carpal tunnel syndrome. *Scandinavian journal of work, environment & health.* 2003;29(3):189-96.

[70] Kwon JY, Kim JY, Hong JT, Sung JH, Son BC, Lee SW. Position Change of the Neurovascular Structures around the Carpal Tunnel with Dynamic Wrist Motion. *Journal of Korean Neurosurgical Society.* 2011;50(4):377-80.

[71] Jarvik JG, Comstock BA, Heagerty PJ, Haynor DR, Fulton-Kehoe D, Kliot M, et al. Magnetic resonance imaging compared with electrodiagnostic studies in patients with suspected carpal tunnel syndrome: predicting symptoms, function, and surgical benefit at 1 year. *Journal of neurosurgery.* 2008;108(3):541-50.

[72] Stabile MJ, Warfield CA. Differential diagnosis of arm pain. *Hospital practice.* 1990;25(1):55-8, 61, 4.

[73] Rehak DC. Pronator syndrome. *Clinics in sports medicine.* 2001;20(3):531-40.

[74] Lee MJ, LaStayo PC. Pronator syndrome and other nerve compressions that mimic carpal tunnel syndrome. *The Journal of orthopaedic and sports physical therapy.* 2004;34(10):601-9.

[75] Carpentier PH. [Raynaud's phenomenon]. *La Revue du praticien.* 2005;55(1):103-7.

[76] Sraj SA, Moussallem CD, Stafford JB. Cubital tunnel syndrome presenting with carpal tunnel symptoms: clinical evidence for sensory ulnar-to-median nerve communication. *American journal of orthopedics.* 2009;38(6):E104-6.

[77] Folberg CR, Weiss AP, Akelman E. Cubital tunnel syndrome. Part I: Presentation and diagnosis. *Orthopaedic review.* 1994;23(2):136-44.

[78] Seradge H, Parker W, Baer C, Mayfield K, Schall L. Conservative treatment of carpal tunnel syndrome: an outcome study of adjunct exercises. *The Journal of the Oklahoma State Medical Association.* 2002;95(1):7-14.

[79] Johnson EW. Splinting vs surgery for carpal tunnel syndrome. JAMA : *the journal of the American Medical Association*. 2003;289(4):420; author reply 1-2.

[80] Dammers JW, Roos Y, Veering MM, Vermeulen M. Injection with methylprednisolone in patients with the carpal tunnel syndrome: a randomised double blind trial testing three different doses. *Journal of neurology*. 2006;253(5):574-7.

[81] Klein RD, Kotsis SV, Chung KC. Open carpal tunnel release using a 1-centimeter incision: technique and outcomes for 104 patients. *Plastic and reconstructive surgery*. 2003;111(5):1616-22.

[82] Badger SA, O'Donnell ME, Sherigar JM, Connolly P, Spence RA. Open carpal tunnel release--still a safe and effective operation. *The Ulster medical journal*. 2008;77(1):22-4.

[83] Brief R, Brief LP. Endoscopic carpal tunnel release: report of 146 cases. The Mount Sinai journal of medicine, New York. 2000;67(4):274-7.

[84] Agee JM, Peimer CA, Pyrek JD, Walsh WE. Endoscopic carpal tunnel release: a prospective study of complications and surgical experience. *The Journal of hand surgery*. 1995;20(2):165-71; discussion 72.

[85] Chow JC. The Chow technique of endoscopic release of the carpal ligament for carpal tunnel syndrome: four years of clinical results. Arthroscopy: the journal of arthroscopic & related surgery : *official publication of the Arthroscopy Association of North America and the International Arthroscopy Association*. 1993;9(3):301-14.

[86] Kuschner SH, Lane CS. Endoscopic versus open carpal tunnel release: big deal or much ado about nothing? *American journal of orthopedics*. 1997;26(9):591-6.

[87] Kasdan ML. Complications of endoscopic and open carpal tunnel release. *The Journal of hand surgery*. 2000;25(1):185.

[88] Palmer AK, Toivonen DA. Complications of endoscopic and open carpal tunnel release. *The Journal of hand surgery*. 1999;24(3):561-5.

[89] Lee DH, Masear VR, Meyer RD, Stevens DM, Colgin S. Endoscopic carpal tunnel release: a cadaveric study. *The Journal of hand surgery*. 1992;17(6):1003-8.

[90] Tanabe T, Okutsu I. An anatomical study of the palmar ligamentous structures of the carpal canal. *Journal of hand surgery*. 1997;22(6):754-7.

[91] Hong JT, Lee SW, Han SH, Son BC, Sung JH, Park CK, et al. Anatomy of neurovascular structures around the carpal tunnel during dynamic

wrist motion for endoscopic carpal tunnel release. *Neurosurgery.* 2006;58(1 Suppl):ONS127-33; discussion ONS-33.

[92] Schwartz JT, Waters PM, Simmons BP. Endoscopic carpal tunnel release: a cadaveric study. Arthroscopy : *the journal of arthroscopic & related surgery : official publication of the Arthroscopy Association of North America and the International Arthroscopy Association.* 1993;9(2):209-13.

[93] Lanz U. Anatomical variations of the median nerve in the carpal tunnel. *The Journal of hand surgery.* 1977;2(1):44-53.

[94] Levy HJ, Soifer TB, Kleinbart FA, Lemak LJ, Bryk E. Endoscopic carpal tunnel release: an anatomic study. Arthroscopy : *the journal of arthroscopic & related surgery : official publication of the Arthroscopy Association of North America and the International Arthroscopy Association.* 1993;9(1):1-4.

[95] Healy C, Watson JD, Longstaff A, Campbell MJ. Magnetic resonance imaging of the carpal tunnel. *Journal of hand surgery.* 1990;15(2):243-8.

[96] Lindau T, Karlsson MK. Complications and outcome in open carpal tunnel release. A 6-year follow-up in 92 patients. *Chirurgie de la main.* 1999;18(2):115-21.

[97] De Smet L. Recurrent carpal tunnel syndrome. Clinical testing indicating incomplete section of the flexor retinaculum. *Journal of hand surgery.* 1993;18(2):189.

[98] Assmus H, Staub F. [Recurrences of carpal tunnel syndrome in long-term haemodialysis patients]. Handchirurgie, Mikrochirurgie, plastische Chirurgie : Organ der Deutschsprachigen Arbeitsgemeinschaft fur Handchirurgie : Organ der Deutschsprachigen Arbeitsgemeinschaft fur Mikrochirurgie der Peripheren Nerven und Gefasse 2005;37(3):158-66.

[99] Stutz N, Gohritz A, van Schoonhoven J, Lanz U. Revision surgery after carpal tunnel release--analysis of the pathology in 200 cases during a 2 year period. *Journal of hand surgery.* 2006;31(1):68-71.

Index

D

E

T